SpringerBriefs in Materials

More information about this series at http://www.springer.com/series/10111

Mykola Borzenkov · Orest Hevus

Surface Active Monomers

Synthesis, Properties, and Application

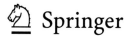 Springer

Mykola Borzenkov
Department of Physics
University of Milano-Bicocca
Milan
Italy

Orest Hevus
Department of Organic Chemistry
Lviv Polytechnic National University
Lviv
Ukraine

ISSN 2192-1091   ISSN 2192-1105   (electronic)
ISBN 978-3-319-08445-9   ISBN 978-3-319-08446-6   (eBook)
DOI 10.1007/978-3-319-08446-6

Library of Congress Control Number: 2014942708

Springer Cham Heidelberg New York Dordrecht London

Printed on acid-free paper

Springer is part of Springer Science+Business Media (www.springer.com)

Preface

The chemistry of surface active monomers is developing very rapidly. Since the first papers devoted to the synthesis and polymerization of surface active monomers were published, numerous researches in this area have been performed. Hence, many reviews highlighting various aspects in the area of surface active monomers were published. The research group at the Department of Organic Chemistry (Lviv Polytechnic National University, Ukraine) has developed its own school dedicated to surface active monomers. In present overview, the most essential information about surface active monomers is summarized. Moreover, the emphasis was made to application of surface active monomers and corresponding surface active polymers for different needs of medicine and biology.

Acknowledgments

Mykola Borzenkov would like to express his gratitude to head of the research group at the Department of Organic Chemistry (Lviv Polytechnic National University) Prof. O. Hevus for his invaluable guidance and support. He is very grateful to Prof. O. Zaichenko and Dr. N. Mitina for their strong assistance and support especially during the investigation of polymerizable properties of synthesized surface active monomers and characterization of resulted polymers. Mykola Borzenkov would like to thank all the current and former members of research group Dr. L. Vuitsyk, Dr. N. Kinash, Dr. A. Kohut, Dr. R. Fleychuk, and Z. Nadashkevich for their cooperation and assistance.

Contents

About the Authors

Mykola Borzenkov received his Ph.D. in Organic Chemistry at Lviv Polytechnic National University, Lviv, Ukraine. The Ph.D. thesis "Synthesis and properties of surface active monomers based on derivatives of hydroxy and amino carboxylic acids" were carried out under supervision of prof. Orest Hevus. At present time M. Borzenkov is a research assistant at Department of Physics at University of Milan-Bicocca (Milan, Italy). His main research fields are synthesis and application of functional surface active monomers, synthesis, functionalization and biomedical application of gold nanoparticles.

Orest Hevus is a professor of Organic Chemistry. From 1979 to the present he has been working at Lviv Polytechnic National University. His research field is synthesis of functional surface active peroxides and monomers.

Introduction

The relevant needs of medicine, biology, and other fields of science and industry in novel polymeric materials possessing a range of "special properties" caused the rapid progress of searching the most efficient ways of their obtaining. The mentioned above "special properties" are following: biocompatibility, controlled distraction stability in living organisms, low toxicity of these materials, and their distraction derivatives etc. Nowadays these polymers are widely utilized as carriers of drugs and genetic materials, biocompatible implants, scaffolds for tissue engineering [1–4]. Customary as a rule corresponding polymeric materials have colloidal structure with functionalized interface. The properties of modern polymer materials are determined not only by chemical structure of polymer but also by the nature of interface and by processes occurred at interface. The presence of various functional groups at the surface of polymeric particles facilitates to perform varied reactions at interface, namely to form implanted polymeric layers with desired properties to immobilize various biomolecules, drugs, luminescent, magnetic, and other markers [5–8]. Hence, the utilization of surface active monomers seems to be a prospective way for synthesis of such polymeric materials.

According to IUPAC definition the classical emulsion polymerization is considered as polymerization whereby monomer(s), initiator, dispersion medium, and colloid stabilizer constitute initially an inhomogeneous system resulting in particles of colloidal dimensions containing the formed polymer. This process involves emulsification of the relatively hydrophobic monomer in water due to the presence of emulsifier, followed by the initiation reaction with either a water-soluble or an oil-soluble free radical initiator. At the end of the process a milky fluid called "polymer dispersion" or "synthetic latex" is formed. This type of polymerization consists of three principal steps, namely initiation, prolongation, and termination. After the emulsion of monomer in aqueous phase and presence of emulsifier micelles ascertained, the polymerization is initiated by the addition of initiator. The free radicals are generated in the aqueous phase and diffuse into monomer-swollen micelles. The corresponding monomer in the micelle polymerizes and the growing chain terminates. At this point the monomer-swollen micelle has turned into a polymer particle. However, this type of polymerization includes some disadvantages, namely connected with the employment of surfactants. Surfactants remain in resulted polymer and it is difficult to completely remove them. Moreover, the utilization of traditional surfactants during emulsion and dispersion polymerization could cause some inconveniences and negatively impacts on properties of resulted polymers. For example, surfactants with low molecular weight can migrate to surface layers of polymers, adversely affecting on adhesion and water resistance. One of the ways of solving these problems is to incorporate the surfactant to a polymer backbone during the polymerization. Therefore, the most reliable strategy is to use surfactants containing unsaturated fragments capable for polymerization and copolymerization with other monomers. Surface active monomers (also are known as surfmers) during the preparation of emulsion of monomers in water are located predominantly on the monomer droplet-water interface thus acting as surfactants stabilizing the emulsion [9]. However, in contrast to traditional surfactants, surfmers due to presence of polymerizable units are incorporated into polymer backbone during the polymerization. The surfmer links due to their surface activity are located predominantly on the surface of polymeric particles providing effective stabilization of the polymer colloid [9]. Such polymer dispersion is considered cleaner, than obtained with non polymerizable surfactants, what is important for biomedical application.

As surfmers locate predominantly at interface during the emulsion polymerization the research of surface active monomers locates at interface of organic, colloidal and polymer chemistry, and results are applied to medicine, pharmacy, and biology. The present survey summarizes the most important information dedicated to the surface active monomers. This review focuses on various techniques of synthesis of surface active monomers with various polymerizable fragments highlighting their surface active properties. Moreover, the polymerization properties of such monomers and synthesis of polymeric materials with units of surfmers is described. Finally, the application of such polymers especially for various fields of biology and medicine is provided.

References

1. George PM, Lyckman AW, LaVan DA et al (2005) Fabrication and biocompatibility of polypyrrole implants suitable for neural prostchetics. Biomaterials 17:3511–3519
2. Liechty WB, Kryscio DR, Slaughter BV, Peppas NA (2010) Polymers for drug delivery systems. Annu Rev Chem Biomol Eng 1:149–173
3. Larson N, Ghandehari H (2012) Polymeric conjugates for drug delivery. Chem Mater 24:840–853
4. Abulateefeh SR, Spain GS, Aylott JW, Chan WC, Garnett MC, Alexander C (2011) Thermoresponsive polymer colloids for drug delivery and cancer therapy. Macromol Biosci 11:1722–1734
5. Pyun J (2007) Nanocomposite materials from functional polymers and magnetic colloids. Polym Rev 47:231–263
6. Sung D, Park S, Jon S (2012) Facile immobilization of biomolecules onto various surfaces using epoxide-containing antibiofouling polymers. Langmuir 28:4507–4514

7. Ho K, Cole N, Chen R, Willcox MD, Rice SA, Kumar N (2012) Immobilization of antibacterial dyhydropyrrol-2-ones on functional polymer supports to prevent bacterial infections in vivo. Antimicrob Agents Chemother 56:1138–1141
8. Shen L (2011) Biocompatible polymer/quantom dots hybrid materials: current status and future developments. J Funct Biomater 2:355–372
9. Nagai K (1994) Polimerization of surface active monomers and applications. Macromol Symp 84:29–36

Chapter 1
Synthesis of Surface Active Monomers

1.1 Basic Concept of Surfmers

As opposite to traditional surfactants, the molecules of surfmers have polymerizable fragments. Therefore, during the polymerization, they act as comonomers and their units are incorporated to the polymer backbone [1]. Application of surfmers containing various functional groups or fragments of compounds of natural origin, displaying essential reactivity during polymerization and surface activity, promotes wide opportunities of obtaining materials with predicted properties. The scheme of emulsion polymerization with application of surfmers is shown in Scheme 1.1. The corresponding scheme illustrates the process of preparation of polymeric dispersions with functionalized surface.

Moreover, the utilization of surfmers during the process of preparation of polymer colloids assures the stability of resulted colloidal systems in wide range of pH and temperature rates [2]. This promotes to obtain the polymeric materials with improved properties.

Nowadays, a wide spectrum of surface-active monomers is synthesized. The chemistry of surfmers till the middle of 1990s is well described in works of Tauer and Guyot [3–5] and in range of other surveys and publications [6–12].

It is worth to mention that modern types of surfmers besides hydrophilic and hydrophobic blocks and polymerizable fragments contain also various functional groups. The presence of corresponding functional groups gives an opportunity to perform different interactions occurring at interface [13, 14]. Copolymerization of functional surfmers results in surface-active copolymers which could be applied as efficient interface modifiers or carriers of biomolecules.

Generically, all surface-active monomers could be classified according to following criteria:

- The function response for surface activity: All surfmers are divided into three main groups: cationic surfmers, anionic surfmers, and nonionic surfmers;

© The Author(s) 2014
M. Borzenkov and O. Hevus, *Surface Active Monomers*,
SpringerBriefs in Materials, DOI: 10.1007/978-3-319-08446-6_1

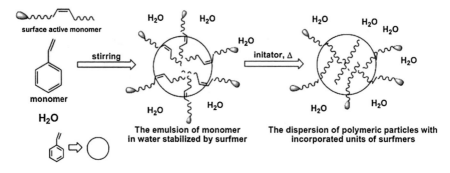

Scheme 1.1 Preparation of polymeric dispersions with functionalized surface

- The type of polymerizable unit: There are following classes of surface-active monomers: maleic surfmers, maleimide-containing surfmers, (meth)acrylic surfmers, and styrenic surfmers (there also exist a range of surfmers with vinyl and allyl polymerizable group, but in current review, we mainly focus on the synthesis of previously mentioned types of surfmers);
- The location of polymerizable fragment in molecule of surfmer: The corresponding fragment could be the terminate substitute either in hydrophilic or hydrophobic part or conjunctive link between these parts;
- The nature and length of hydrophobic blocks and origin of hydrophilic moieties, and the presence of functional groups.

The general structure of surface-active monomers could be illustrated with Scheme 1.2.

The detailed description of above-mentioned classification is provided.

Anionic surfmers generally contains carboxylate, sulfonate, and phosphate moieties. Surface-active monomers with carboxylic groups are known to be prospective compounds for creation of anionic surface-active copolymers applied for drug delivery as well as for binding of peptides and amino acids [15]. The cationic surfmers containing the fragments of amines or tetraalkylammonium salts are widely applied [16]. Moreover, these compounds manifest antibactericidal properties and surfmers containing quaternary ammonium fragment or zwitterionic

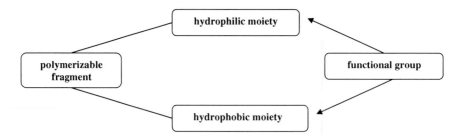

Scheme 1.2 General structure of surface-active monomers

function are the promising reagents for creation of modifiers of negative-charged surfaces [17]. Moreover, cationic oligomers based on above-mentioned surfmers provide efficient protein-binding facilities and can be used as carriers for nucleic acids, polypeptides, as well as some pharmaceutical substances [18]. Nonionic surfmers dissolve in water without ionization and in principal contain long poly(ethylene oxide) blocks [15].

The polymerization capability of such compounds as in case of typical monomers is determined by the nature of polymerizable fragment [19]. Diesters of maleic acid were one of the first types of synthesized surface-active monomers [15]. The main singularity of these surfmers is that the fragment of maleic acid acts as conjunctive link between hydrophilic and hydrophobic parts of surfmer. As classical maleic monomers, the corresponding monomers are not able to homopolymerize [19]. During the copolymerization with other monomers, they form alternating copolymers [20]. Moreover, the insertion of substitutes of different nature and in various combinations in their molecules allows regulating the colloidal properties of monomers in a wide range. Copolymerization of (meth)acrylic surface-active monomers allows to obtain non-toxic, elastic (in case of acrylates) polymers with high adhesion. Therefore, they could be applied as drug delivery vehicles [21] or surface modificators [22]. The application of surface-active monomers for obtaining the functionalized polymers via miniemulsion polymerization is well highlighted in a review of Craspy and Lanfester [23].

As it was told previously, the polymerizable part in the molecule of surfmer could be located either in hydrophilic part or in hydrophobic part or between these two parts. However, the position of C=C bond in the molecule of surface-active monomer has considerable impacts on properties of resulted copolymers [24].

The nature of hydrophilic and hydrophobic parts plays an important role and appreciably impacts the behavior of surface-active monomer [24]. Variation of length and origin of liphophilic and hydrophilic fragments allows to tailor hydrophilic–liphophilic balance of surfmer and its preferential location in colloid system [11]. Furthermore, the nature of lipophilic fragment of surfmer provides the affinity to different surfaces.

Besides the surface-active monomers with traditional diblock structure, it is worth to mention surfmers with alternately located liphophilic and hydrophilic blocks. The oligoesters of dicarboxylic acids and poly(ethylene glycols) with different molecular weights and terminated polymerizable fragments are glaring examples of corresponding types of surfmers. The singularity of these monomers is that they are capable of reversibly responding to changes of polarity of environment, providing the stability of colloidal systems [25].

Combination of type of surface activity, nature of liphophilic moiety, and the position of polymerizable fragment promotes solving numerous problems connecting with further development and modification of polymeric layers located on interface of colloidal systems.

During last years, more attention is focused on development of surface-active monomers containing the fragments of compounds of nature origin, namely cholesterol, saccharides, peptides, and lipids.

Scheme 1.3 General structure of saccharide-containing monomers

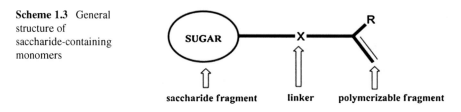

saccharide fragment   linker   polymerizable fragment

The range of papers devoted to the synthesis of novel saccharide-containing monomers was published [26–31]. Nowadays, saccharide-containing monomers especially surface-active monomers are widely applied for obtaining polymers of biomedical application [32]. One of the most common models of saccharide surfmers contains liphophilic and polymerizable fragments which are the substitutes of glucoside hydroxyl. The general structure of these monomers is shown in Scheme 1.3.

The surface-active monomers which are the analogs of lecithin were synthesized, and their properties were described [33]. These monomers are capable of reverse processing of copolymerization–decopolymerization. Moreover, the S–S bonds of resulted polymers have the same nature as S–S bonds in the molecules of proteins. Also a great attention is focused on synthesis of surfmers, the analogous or derivatives of phosphoglycerides which are known to be the typical structural lipids of biological membranes [34]. The corresponding compounds are applied for modification of various polymeric scaffolds following with formation of lipophilic layer. The synthesis and application of surfmers containing peptide fragments are also highlighted [35–38].

The obtaining and application of surface-active monomers for creation of polymeric monolayers and liposomes are described in reviews of Ringsdorf et al. [39, 40]. The monograph of Zaicev [41] is dedicated to synthesis and properties of surface-active monomers for creation of ultrathin oriented membranes of biomedical application.

The surface-active initiators (inisurf) are considered to be an attractive class of surfactants due to the capability of generation of radicals. The corresponding compounds contain hydrophilic and hydrophobic parts as well as a functional group capable of generating radicals, either azo- or peroxy group [24]. The inisurf can be either low molecular weight or polymer substances and contain one or multiple reactive radical-generating groups. As a typical surfactant, inisurfs have either ionic or nonionic nature of hydrophilic moiety. The hydrophobic part of inisurf in most cases consists of alkyl, alkylphenol, and poly(propylene oxide) fragments. The surface activity of surface-active initiators is known to be the most important parameter that significantly impacts polymerization process. These compounds are used for functionalization followed with further modification of interface of colloidal systems. The main advantage of surface-active initiators is focused on the possibility of utilization of lower amount of components (monomer, water) during the emulsion or dispersion polymerization. The wide range of papers summarizing the investigations in the field of surface-active initiators was published previously [42–47].

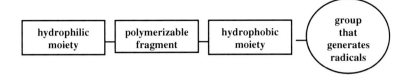

Scheme 1.4   The structure of molecule of peroxide-containing surfmer

As a result of investigations in this field, the new class of surface-active monomers, namely surface-active monomers–initiators or peroxide-containing surfmers, was established. The structure of molecule of peroxide-containing surfmer is shown in Scheme 1.4.

Synthesis of surfmers containing di-tertial-peroxide groups in liphophilic moiety was reported [24, 48]. The application of peroxide-containing surfmers during the emulsion and dispersion polymerization provides the immobilization of peroxide groups onto the surface of polymeric particles directly during their formation. This allows to perform various polymer-analogous transformations by free radical reactions due to the presence of peroxide groups on the surface. Also, the main advantage of employment of peroxide-containing surfmers during emulsion polymerization is that in this case, the corresponding surfmer acts as emulsifier, comonomer, and initiator of polymerization at the same time. Therefore, as opposite to classical emulsion polymerization, the additional presence of emulsifier and initiator is not required.

The synthesis of surfmers with various hydrophilic and hydrophobic moieties and with different nature of polymerizable fragments is described in following subchapters.

1.2 Synthesis of Maleic Surfmers

Within different types of surfmers, special attention is paid to the ways of obtaining of surface-active maleates. It has been already mentioned above that the main singularity of these monomers is that they are almost incapable of homopolymerization and generally can form alternate copolymers. The general structure of this class of surfmers is shown in Scheme 1.5.

Such maleic surfmers could be easily synthesized utilizing maleic anhydride, aliphatic alcohols (as hydrophobic moiety), and compounds responsible for formation of hydrophilic moieties (PEG, propanesultone, aminoethanol and its derivatives, etc.) [16, 24]. Acylation of aliphatic alcohols leads to formation of intermediate monoalkyl maleates. The hydrophobic constituent is incorporated to the reaction of carboxylic group. However, the employment of poly(ethylene glycols) of different molecular weights for these purposes could be a problematic because of using a fivefold excess of PEG with subsequent removing of the excess

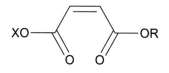

Scheme 1.5 General structure of maleic surfmers. R and X are hydrophilic and hydrophobic moieties correspondingly

Scheme 1.6 The cationic maleate surfmer synthesized from corresponding dialkylmaleate

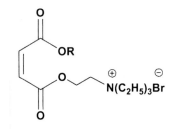

of poly(ethylene glycol) from reaction media. The application of monosubstituted derivatives such as poly(ethylene glycol) methyl ether with different molecular weights is more convenient [24].

One of the representatives of these monomers was synthesized by subsequent reaction of maleic anhydride with aliphatic alcohols C_{12}–C_{18} and propanesultone [3]. Other types of cationic maleate surfmers were synthesized in several steps [49, 50]. Thus, the intermediate ester was synthesized by reaction of maleic anhydride with aliphatic alcohols. The corresponding maleate was subjected to O-alkylation, which resulted in formation of proper dialkylmaleate. For better solubility in water, the resulted dialkylmaleate was quaternized using different alkylating agents. The chemical structure of one of these surface-active monomers is shown in Scheme 1.6.

Also it is necessary to mention the maleate surfmers synthesized by interaction of monoalkyl maleates with glycidyl trimethylammonium chloride [51] as it is shown in Scheme 1.7.

Surface-active maleate monomer was synthesized from maleic anhydride, polyoxoethylene esters of fatty alcohols and sodium hydroxide as it was described [52]. The synthesis conditions and the colloidal properties of resulted monomer were studied. Youshimura et al. [53] prepared telomeric anionic compounds by performing an interaction of maleic anhydride with aliphatic alcohols followed with further telomerization in the presence of alkanethiol. Amphoteric surfmer was synthesized by reaction of 2-hydroxy-N,N,N-trimethylammonium-chloride with monoalkyl maleates C_8–C_{12} in the presence of basic catalysis [54]. Cationic maleic dialkyl surfmer containing 12 atoms of carbon in hydrophobic part was synthesized and applied for emulsion copolymerization with other monomers [55].

The synthesis of reactive fumaric-, maleic-, and itaconic surface-active monomers with both fluorine-containing groups and hydrophilic groups was reported in US patent published in 2009 [56]. Monofluorooctyl surface-active maleate was synthesized and applied for radical polymerization in miniemulsions [57].

Scheme 1.7 Interaction of monoalkylmaleates with glycidyl trimethylammonium chloride

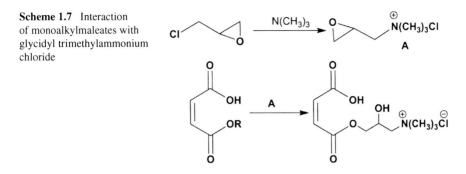

The synthesis of reactive anionic maleic surfmer containing hydrophobic oligosyloxane chain was reported [2]. The range of maleate surfmers were synthesized by reaction of maleic isoimides containing long alkylic chains with hydrophilic derivatives of amines [58]. Another type of maleic surfmer was synthesized by interaction of maleic anhydride, PEG, and phthalic anhydride [59].

An extensive range of maleic surface-active monomers with hydrophilic polyethylene glycolic, propanesultonic, or triethylamine moieties and hydrophobic alkylic, fluoroalkylic, oligomethylsiloxanic, and saccharide moieties were prepared by the research group at the Department of Organic Chemistry of Lviv Polytechnic National University (Lviv, Ukraine) [16, 24, 60–63]. Moreover, the derivatives of these monomers containing peroxide groups and other functions such as phosphate group were obtained. The corresponding peroxide-containing surface-active maleates consisted of mono(ω-peroxyalkyl)maleates as hydrophobic moieties and of hydrophilic polyethylene glycolic, carboxylate, propanesultonic, or triethylamine moieties [48]. The saccharide surfmers were synthesized utilizing diisopropilidengalactose, maleic anhydride, propanesultone, and PEG monomethyl ether as initial compounds. The chemical structures of some of these mentioned monomers are shown in the Scheme 1.8.

However, the application of copolymer family containing di-tert-peroxide peroxide for initiation of polymerization from the surface is limited due to high thermal stability of peroxide group. The surfmers with peroxyester groups are more promising for creating surface functionalized polymeric colloids due to their lower thermal stability.

For this purpose, another interesting approach in the preparation of functional surfmers was developed by the scientists from mentioned research group. Surface-active monomers that have polymerizable group and a functional group separated from each other via spacers of different length and nature are interesting prospects for developing of novel types of surface-active copolymers. Various fragments of bifunctional compounds (diols, dicarboxylic acids, diamines, etc.) that are used as spacers could be incorporated into surfmer structure via successive interaction due to their functional groups. However, selective transformation of one of the two equally reactive functional groups is quite problematic. As a result, the final product contains impurities of bifunctional derivatives, which is a serious issue in monomer synthesis. Such problems can be omitted by using various heterocyclic reagents (oxyranes, lactones, sultones, etc.) since they are known to selectively form monosubstituted

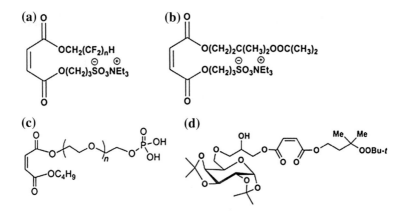

Scheme 1.8   Chemical structures of synthesized novel surface-active maleates

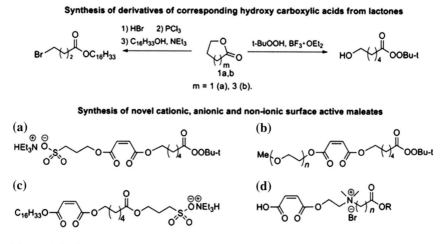

Scheme 1.9   The chemical structures of surface-active maleates synthesized from lactones of ω-hydroxy carboxylic acids

derivatives in ring-opening reactions in mild conditions [64]. Lactones of corresponding carboxylic acids are particularly promising reagents for incorporation of hydrophobic spacers. The utilization of lactones of different carboxylic acids and with various ring sizes allows varying hydrophilic–lipophilic balance and the position of polymerizable fragment relative to the other functional groups in molecule of surfmer. Hence, the novel surface-active monomers containing poly(ethylene glycol), carboxylic, sulfonate, and quaternary ammonium hydrophilic fragments and tert-butylperoxy groups utilizing lactones of ω-hydroxycarboxtlic acids as initial materials were synthesized [65, 66]. The chemical structures of maleate surfmers synthesized are displayed in Scheme 1.9.

A new bifunctional maleic surfmer was prepared by reacting polyoxyethylene 4-nonyl-2-propylene-phenol nonionic reactive surfactant with maleic anhydride followed by esterification with poly(ethylene glycol) [67].

Also the monomers containing maleimide fragment should be also mentioned. Maleimide and its derivatives are prepared from maleic anhydride by treatment with amines followed by dehydration [68]. Due the some special properties of maleimide fragment, these compounds are successfully applied in polymer chemistry, biology, and medicine for solving a number of important tasks. Hence, a very short description of corresponding compounds is provided in Sect. 1.3.

1.3 Synthesis of Surface-Active Monomers Containing Maleimide Fragment

Nowadays, maleimide monomers are widely used in medicine and biotechnology. Meleimides are known to be good dienophiles, and they are almost incapable of homopolymerization. The derivatives of maleimides could be utilized as agents for regulation of inner cell adhesion of molecules [69]. These compounds are capable for polymerization in the presence of peroxides or under UV irradiation. Moreover, maleimides and maleimide-containing monomers as Michael acceptors are favorable compounds for binding of thiol groups forming stable thioether bonds [70]. The reaction of maleimides with thiols is considered as one of the best known site-specific, simple, and quantitative protein modification reaction. This process is displayed in Scheme 1.10.

The corresponding compounds are utilized in biology for studying the structure of proteins. Generally, for these purposes, the labeling of proteins with maleimide-containing fluorescent compounds is performed [71].

The synthesis techniques of various maleimido carboxylic acids and their derivatives were reported in 1970s. Particularly, the works of Rich et al. [72] Skrifvars, and Schmidt [73] should be noticed.

Maleimide groups are used to facilitate covalent attachment of proteins and other molecules to polymers [74]. The application of graft-meleimide surfactants allowed to perform efficient functionalization of lipid nanoparticles. Special attention is focused on synthesis of maleimide derivatives containing PEG fragments due to the fact that PEGylation became an attractive technique for monitoring of release, biodistribution, toxicology of drugs, and proteins. Accordingly, numerous papers describing various approaches in this field could be found. Many preparation techniques of PEG maleimides involve connecting an activated PEG to a small linker molecule comprising a maleimide group; many of which are available commercially [75]. For this reason, the brief overview regarding the poly(ethylene glycol)-containing maleimide monomer is provided.

The reaction of phenylisocyanate with the hydroxyl group of monomethoxy-PEG (mPEG) was developed as a platfrom for synthesis of desired PEG reagents [74]. A wide spectrum of PEGylated maleimide monomers was synthesized based

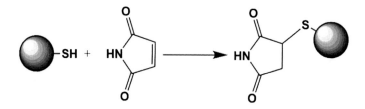

Scheme 1.10 The capability of maleimides of binding thiol groups

on monomethoxy-PEG, and their properties were described [76–79]. The application of PEGylated maleimides for the modification of hemoglobin was studied in detail by the scientists from University of Florida [80]. Novel surface-active monomer distearyl-phosphatidyl–ethanilamino-PEG$_{5000}$-maleimide was synthesized and successfully applied for design of efficient carriers of the drugs [81]. The properties of photon-upconverting nanoparticles decorated with surface-active maleimide–PEG–COOH are reported in paper published in 2012 [82].

Also it is worth to mention in a few words about the protection of the reactive maleimide double bond prior to polymerization. This approach provides the synthesis of novel monomers containing a masked maleimide [83]. The resulted polymers contain protected reactive maleimide groups on their side chains. Diels–Alder reaction between furan and maleimide was adapted for the protection of the reactive maleimide double bond prior to polymerization [84]. Upon heating, a retro Diels–Alder reaction takes place and the blocked maleimide group becomes unblocked. The process is illustrated in Scheme 1.11.

The synthesis of novel monomers bearing protected maleimide group for the preparation of latex particles including those having active maleimide surface groups was claimed in US patent published in 2011 [85]. In this patent, the synthesis of corresponding monomers using furan-protected maleimide, bromo alcohols, acryloyl chloride, and vinylbenzoic esters as initial compounds is described. Accordingly, the protection of maleimide group provides an opportunity to synthesize monomers containing various polymerizable fragments and masked maleimide group.

Two optically active maleimide monomers containing cholesteryl groups were synthesized and applied as comonomers during copolymerization with styrene [86]. Synthesized graft-maleimide surfactants promoted the functionalization of lipid nanoparticles [87]. The synthesis of functional maleimide monomers based on 4-maleimido benzoic acid was reported in paper published in 2002 [88]. Two new surfactant molecules containing thermally labile Diels–Alder adducts connecting the hydrophilic and hydrophobic sections of each molecule were reported [89]. These two surfactants possess identical hydrophobic dodecyl tail segments and have phenol and carboxylic acid hydrophilic headgroups, respectively. Synthesis of maleimide-terminated aryl ether sulfone oligomers and copolymerization with divinylbenzene was reported in a paper published recently in Advances in Science and Technology [90].

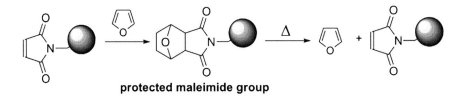

protected maleimide group

Scheme 1.11 The protection of maleimide group via Diels–Alder reaction

Scheme 1.12 The chemical structure of sodium 9(and 10)-acrylamidostearate

$$CH_2=CH-C \underset{NH-CH-(CH_2)_{7(8)}COONa}{\overset{O}{\diagup}} \quad (CH_2)_{7(8)}CH_3$$

1.4 Synthesis of (Meth)acrylate Surface-Active Monomers

In present subchapter, the overview of synthesis of (meth)acrylate surface-active monomers is provided. It has already been mentioned previously that due to the set of important properties, the poly(meth)acrylate monomers are considered as attractive prospects for application in various fields including biomedical application. Hence, the synthesis of initial (meth)acrylate monomers especially surface-active seems to be an important task.

One of the early representatives of corresponding monomers was sodium 9(and 10)-acrylamidostearate that was synthesized for preparation of styrene-butadiene latexes [91]. The chemical structure of these surfmer is shown in Scheme 1.12.

Juang and Krieger [92] synthesized sulfopropylmethacrylate monomer

$$CH_2=C(CH_3)-C(O)-O-CH_2-CH_2-CH_2-SO_3Na$$

and applied this monomer for preparation of polystyrene latexes.

In the paper published in 1991, the synthesis and application of anionic surface-active monomers is reported [93]. The chemical structures of these monomers are displayed in Scheme 1.13.

The acylation of corresponding groups in hydrophilic moieties of synthetic or nature origin surfactants with acryloyl or methacryloyl chlorides is considered to be one of the most simple and convenient ways of synthesis of proper surface-active monomers [94]. For example, the acylation of primary amine group of octadecylamine and phosphatidylethanolamines allows to synthesize conformable monomers with high yields [95]. For synthesis of surfmers containing polymerizable fragment in aliphatic part, the acylation with acryloyl or methacryloyl chlorides of hydroxyl groups of hydroxy carboxylic acids with different chain length was applied [96]. Thus, for example, the acylation of hydroxy groups of 12-hydroxydodecanoic acid and 16-hydroxyhexadecanoic acids led to formation of corresponding derivatives [97, 98].

Scheme 1.13 Chemical structures of previously synthesized anionic surfmers

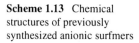

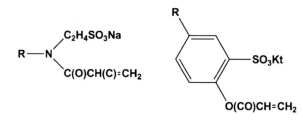

It has been already mentioned that the acylation of hydroxyl or amino groups with acryloyl or methacryloyl chlorides provides a wide opportunity to create the surfmers with terminated polymerizable fragment located either in hydrophilic or hydrophobic part. Sometimes, introduction of the quarternary ammonium fragment or residue of phosphoric acid in the structure of corresponding monomers is performed. Novel types of surface-active monomers were synthesized by acylation of hydroxyl groups of one or both fatty aliphatic chains of lipids with acryloyl or methacryloyl chloride [99]. Moreover, the acylation of hydroxyl or amino groups with acryloyl or methacryloyl chlorides of molecules of surfactants is applied in organic chemistry for synthesis of lipid-like monomers for modification of proteins [100]. This provides the facility not only to immobilize the membrane-active compounds in polymeric membranes but also to perform the copolymerization with polymeric surroundings [101].

The cationic surface-active monomers were synthesized by acylation of ω-dialkylaminoalcohols with methacryloyl chloride followed with quaternization with benzyl chloride [102]. Macromonomers, containing alternate hydrophilic and hydrophobic moieties, were synthesized by polycondensation of aliphatic dicarboxylic acids with PEGs followed with subsequent acylation with methacryloyl chloride [24].

The saccharide containing functional acrylate monomers [31] were synthesized according to the Scheme 1.14 illustrated.

The incorporation of various hydrophilic and hydrophobic groups due to the presence of functional groups provides the opportunities of tailoring the surfactant properties in a wide range.

Black et al. [103] reported the synthesis of monomer obtained by acylation of di-O-isopropylidene-α-D-glucofuranose with methacryloyl chloride. The synthesis of methacrylate sugar containing monomers and their polymerization properties were reported in a paper published in Biomacromolecules in 2003 [104].

At the department of Organic Chemistry of Lviv Polytechnic National University, the saccharide-containing acrylate and methacrylate monomers were synthesized utilizing di-isopropylidene hexoses as initial compounds. The resulted monomers contained the polymerizable fragment directly near atom C_6 or separated from C_6 via glycerin spacer [60].

Other types of methacrylate surface-active monomers containing poly(ethylene glycol) hydrophobic blocks and phosphate groups were synthesized by the same research group [105]. The structures of corresponding monomers are shown in Scheme 1.15.

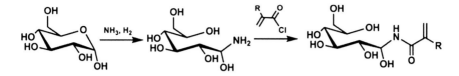

Scheme 1.14   Synthesis of saccharide-containing functional monomers by reductive amination of aldehyde group of hexose

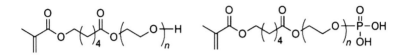

Scheme 1.15   Novel type of nonionic methacrylate surfmer and its phosphate derivative

Scheme 1.16   The structure of 2-(ω-phosphonooxy-2-oxaalkyl)acrylate monomers

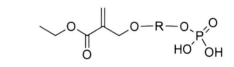

Klee and Lehmann [106] reported about the synthesis of novel stable to hydrolysis surface-active 2-(ω-phosphonooxy-2-oxaalkyl)acrylate monomers for self-etching and self-priming one part adhesive. These monomers were synthesized in three steps, and their structure is shown in Scheme 1.16.

A range of hydrophilic and lipophilic polyfunctional acrylate monomers and oligomers were synthesized based on the condensation reaction of aldehydes with acrylates [107]. The acrylate monomer with long hydrophobic alkylic chain was synthesized by reaction of hydroxyethyl acrylate with methyl oleate by scientists from Republic of Korea [108]. Another hydrophobic monomer, namely 2-octyl-dodecyl acrylate, was synthesized, and its properties were studied [109]. The synthesis of cationic metacrylate monomer containing relatively long alkylic chain, namely 11-(methacryloyloxo)-undecyl(trymethylammonium) bromide, was reported in a paper published in 2011 [110]. The chemical structure of corresponding monomer is shown in Scheme 1.17.

The scientist from Great Britain synthesized a range of surface-active (meth) acrylates containing quaternary ammonium fragments [111]. The colloidal properties and polymerizable properties below and higher critical micelle concentration (CCM) were studied.

The synthesis of surface-active metacrylic monomer (methacryloyl ethylendioxycarbonyl)benzyl *N,N*-dithiocarbamate was described in paper published in 2002 [112]. The reported monomer was applied in surface photografting on crosslinked polymer substrates. The synthesis of surface-active sodium methyl(11-methacryloyloxyundecyl)phosphonate is described in the paper published in 2004

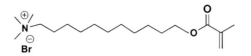

Scheme 1.17 Chemical structure of synthesized 11-(methacryloyloxy)-undecyl (trymethyl-ammonium) bromide

[113]. Thomas et al. [114] reported about synthesis of perfluoroalkylethyl methacrylate and surface-active polymers based on obtained monomers. Ishihara et al. [115] synthesized a methacrylic monomer containing phospholipid polar functional group for creation of the structure of cell membrane. It was has been already told that monomers containing phospholipid groups were successfully applied for binding of biomolecules. Therefore, a functional monomer n-nitrophenylox ycarbonyl(oxyethylene) methacrylte with active ester group was obtained [116]. The copolymerization of the synthesized monomer with methacryloxyethyl phosphorylcholine led to formation of phospholipid polymer.

Senhaj et al. [117] reported about the preparation of surface-active methacrylic phosphonated monomer, namely sodium methyl(11-methacryloyloxyundecyl) phosphonate. This monomer was synthesized in several stages.

Novel surface-active monomer was synthesized by subsequent reactions of cumylsuccinic anhydride with poly(propylene glycol)acrylate, 1,3-propanesultone and tryethylamine [118]. The synthesis of novel bis(methacrylates) with cholesteryl group was reported in recently published paper [119]. A series of polymerizable quaternary ammonium compounds were synthesized with the aim of using them in methacrylate dental composites [120]. The corresponding monomers were formed by reaction of polymerizable amine with different commercial alkyl iodides through Menschutkin reaction.

The synthesis of a range of surfmers with terminal acrylate group on the hydrophilic moiety was reported in a recently published paper [121]. The prepared surfmers were classified into three groups according to hydrophobic chain lengths: the first group was single tailed with different hydrophobic chain lengths; the second group was asymmetric double tailed—one of them was dodecenyl, and the other is octyl or tetradecyl or octadecyl from fatty alcohols—and the third was symmetric double tailed. A novel polymerizable anionic gemini surfactant containing two anionic monomeric parts linked with an ethylene spacer and polymerizable methacryloxy groups covalently bound to the terminal of the hydrocarbon chains was synthesized, and the physicochemical properties in aqueous solution and polymerizable properties were studied [122]. The paper published in 2014 was devoted to novel anionic polymerizable surfactant sodium (5-acryloyl-2-(dodecyloxy)phenyl) methane sulfonate synthesized from phenol, acrylic acid, and bromododecane by esterification, Frise rearrangement, sulfomethylation reaction, and Williamson etherification [123].

Scheme 1.18   Chemical
structure of anionic surfmer
synthesized by S.R. Tsaur
and R.M. Fitch

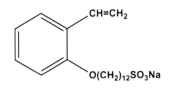

1.5   Synthesis of Surface-Active Monomers Containing Styrene Polymerizable Fragments

The diblock poly(ethylene oxide)-poly(propylene oxide) macromonomers with styrene fragment located in the end of hydrophobic part were synthesized and applied in emulsion polymerization [124].

In the paper published in *Macromolecules* in 1998, the techniques of synthesis of styrene macromonomers containing terminated aldehyde and acetal functional groups are described [125].

The synthesis of styrene-containing macromonomers with general structure

$$H_3C-O-(CH_2CH_2O)_n-(CH_2)_m-C_6H_4-CH=CH_2$$

was reported in the paper published at the beginning of 1990s [126].

The styrene monomers containing hydrophilic PEG chains and hydrophobick alkylik blocks were synthesized [127]. The impact of lengths of these two moieties on colloidal properties was also studied.

Tsaur and Fitch [11] reported the synthesis and properties of anionic styrene surfmer. The structure of corresponding surfmer is shown in Scheme 1.18.

In the paper of Soula et al. [128] published in 1993, the synthesis and application of anionic surfmer with terminated polymerizable fragment is described. At the Department of Organic Chemistry of Lviv Polytechnic National University, the quaternization of tertial aliphatic amines with *n*-chloromethyl styrene led to formation of cationic surfmers [24]. The structure of mentioned surfmers is shown in Scheme 1.19.

Also it is worth to mention about styrene monomers containing saccharide fragments. Preliminary oxidation of glucopiranose to lactone of gluconic acid followed with interaction with 4-aminosryrene led to formation of corresponding saccharide monomer [129] (Scheme 1.20).

A range of saccharide containing monomers with styrene fragments were synthesized from diisopropylidenegalactose via Grigand reaction [130]. Novel saccharide monomers containing styrene fragment were synthesized by O-alkylation of derivatives of galaktopiranose and glukofuranoze with 4-chloromethyl styrene [60]. Another type of saccharide monomers was synthesized by subsequent reactions of diisopropilidengalactose with epichlorohydrin, *N,N*-dimethylaminohexanoic acid, and 4-chloromethyl styrene [65, 131].

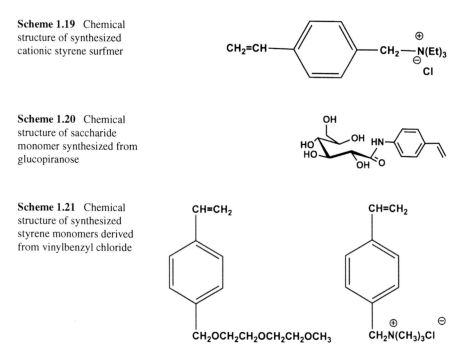

Scheme 1.19 Chemical structure of synthesized cationic styrene surfmer

Scheme 1.20 Chemical structure of saccharide monomer synthesized from glucopiranose

Scheme 1.21 Chemical structure of synthesized styrene monomers derived from vinylbenzyl chloride

Nagasaki et al. [132] reported about the synthesis of novel functional styrene monomers having trimethylsilyl and hidroxyalkyl groups by the reaction between 4-vinylbenzyllithium derivatives and oxiranes. The synthesis of styrene monomers based on vinylbenzyl chloride was reported [133]. The chemical structure of these monomers is shown in Scheme 1.21

A series of tail-type cationic surface-active monomers with the cationic charge at the ω-end and styrenic polymerizable fragment were synthesized as a novel cationic polymerizable surfactant [134].

Summarizing the chapter one, it should be said that due to rapid development of novel materials of biomedical application, synthesis of surface-active monomers is still important task of organic chemistry. Therefore, a general characterization of surface-active monomers and a brief review of synthesis of these compounds with different polymerizable fragments have been performed. The next chapter focuses on colloidal properties of surface-active monomers.

References

1. Ottewill RH, Satgurunathan R (1988) Non-ionic lattices in aqueous media. Part 2. Stability to add electrolytes. J Colloid Polym Sci 266:543–547
2. Capek I (2000) Surface active properties of polyoxyethylene macromonomers and their role in radical polymerization in disperse systems. Adv Colloid Interface Sci 88:295–357

3. Guyot A, Tauer K (1994) Reactive surfactants in emulsion polymerization. Adv Polym Sci 111:43–65

4. Tauer K, Goebel KH, Kosmella S et al (1988) Neuere Entwicklungen bei der Synthese von Polymerdispersionen. Plaste Kautschuk 35:373–378

5. Tauer K, Goebel KH, Kosmella S et al (1990) Emulsion polymerization in the presence of polymerizable emulsifiers and surface active initiators. Makromol Chem, Macromol Symp 31:107–121

6. Holmberg K (1992) Polymerizable surfactants. Prog Org Coat 20:235–241

7. Nagai K (1996) Radical polymerization and potential applications of surface-active monomers. Trends Polym Sci 4:122–126

8. Asua JM, Schoonbrood HA (1998) Reactive surfactants in heterophase polymerization. Acta Polym 49:671–686

9. Holmberg K (1998) Novel Surfactants: Preparation, Applications, and Biodegradability. Marcell Dekker, New York

10. Asua JM (1997) Polymeric Dispersions: Principles and Applications. Kluwer Academic Publishers, Dordrecht

11. Tsaur SL, Fitch RM (1987) Preparation and properties of polystyrene model: I. Preparation of surface active monomers and model colloids derived therefrom. J Colloid Interface Sci 115:450–462

12. Laschewsky A (1995) Molecular concepts, self-organisation and properties of polysoaps. Adv Polym Sci 124:59–86

13. Borzenkov M et al (2011) The obtaining of functional surface-active monomers based on tert-butylperoxy-6-hydroxyhexanoate. Chem Chem Technol 5:363–366

14. Busci A, Forkada J, Gibanel S (1998) Monodisperse polysterene latex particles functionalized by the macromonomer technique. Macromolecules 31:581–620

15. Dahlgren AG, Claesson PM, Audebert R (1994) Highly charged cationic polyelectrolytes on mica: influence of polyelectrolyte concentration on surface forces. J Colloid Interface Sci 166:343–349

16. Kohut AM (2006) Sintez i vlastuvosti poverhnevo-aktuvnuh monomeriv i peroxydiv (Synthesis and properties of surface active monomers and peroxides). Dissertation, Lviv Polytechnic National University

17. O'Donell J, Schumacher GE, Antonucci JM, Skrtic D (2009) Structure-composition-property relationships in polymeric amorphous calcium phosphate-based dental composites. Materials 2:1929–1954

18. Tang MX, Szoka FC (1997) The influence of polymer structure on the interactions of cationic polymers with DNA and morphology of the resulting complexes. Gene Ther 8:823–832

19. Hevus O, Kohut A, Fleychuk R, Zaichenko A, Pashinnik V, Shermolovich Y (2007) Novel surface active maleate monomers for obtaining non–emulsified latexes. React Eng 2:F5–F6

20. Weiss P, Gerecht JF, Krems IJ (1959) Graft copolymers from poly(styrene co dimethyl maleate) and poly(styrene co allyl acetate). J Polym Sci 35:343–354

21. Zaichenko O, Mitina N et al (2010) Oligoperoxide based physically detectable nanocomposites for cell targeting, visualization and treatment. In: AIP Conference Proceedings, vol 1275, pp 178–182

22. Zaichenko O et al (2008) Novel functional nanoscale composites on the basis of oligoperoxide surfactants: syntheses and biomedical applications. Biotechnology 1:82–94

23. Craspy D, Landfester K (2010) Miniemulsion polymerization as a versatile tool for the synthesis of functionalized polymers. Beilstein J Org Chem 6:1132–1148

24. Hevus OI (2010) Funkcionalni poverhnevo-aktuvni peroxydy I monomery yak reagentu dlia oderjannia reakciynozdatnuh modufikatoriv poverhni (Functional surface active peroxides and monomers for creation of reactive surface modifiers). Dissertation, Lviv Polytechnic National University

25. Voronov A, Kohut A et al (2006) Invertible architectures from amphiphilic polyesters. Langmuir 22:1946–1948

26. Boysen M (2007) Carbohydrates as synthetic tools in organic chemistry. Chem Eur J 13:8648–8659
27. Ohnol K, Fukuda T, Kitano H (1998) Free radical polymerization of a sugar residue-carrying styryl monomer with a lipophilic alkoxyamine initiator: synthesis of a well-defined novel glycolipid. Macromol Chem Phys 199:2193–2197
28. Jutz O et al (2005) Synthesis of hyperbranched glycopolymers via self-condensing atom transfer radical copolymerization of a sugar-carrying acrylate. Macromolecules 9:38
29. Wang Q, Dordick JS, Linhardt RJ (2002) Synthesis and application of carbohydrate-containing polymers. Chem Mater 14:3232–3244
30. Stanek LG, Heilmann SM, Gleason WB (2006) Preparation and copolymerization of a novel carbohydrate containing monomer. Carbohydr Polym 65:552–556
31. Narain R, Jhury D (2002) Synthesis and polymerization of novel vinylgluconamides. Polym Int 51:85
32. Narain R (ed) (2011) Engineered Carbohydrate-Based Materials for Biomedical Applications: Polymers, Surfaces, Dendrimers, Nanoparticles, and Hydrogels. Wiley, Hoboken
33. Regene SL et al (1983) Polymerized-depolymerized vesicles. A reversible phosphatidylcholine-based membrane. J Am Chem Soc 105:6354–6355
34. Birdi KS (1989) Lipid and Biopolymer Monolayers at Liquid Interfaces. Plenum Press, London
35. Fendler JH (1982) Membrane Mimetic Chemistry: Characterization and Applications of Micelles, Microemulsions, Monolayers, Bilayers, Vesicles, Host–Guest Systems and Polyions. Wiley, New York
36. Huges SR et al (1996) Two-hybrid system as a model to study the interaction of β-amyloid peptide monomers. Proc Natl Acad Sci USA 93:2065–2070
37. Yamin R et al (2009) Acyl peptide hydrolase degrades monomeric and oligomeric amyloid-beta peptide. Mol Neurodegeneration 4:33
38. Haeshin L, Park TG (2003) A novel method for indentifying PEGylation sites of protein using boitinylated PEG derivatives. J Pharm Sci 93:97–103
39. Ringsdorf J et al (1990) Specific interactions of proteins with functional lipid monolayers—ways of simulating biomembrane process. Angew Chem 29:1269–1285
40. Gros L, Ringsdorf J, Schupp H (1981) Polymere modellmemmbranen. Angew Chem 93:105–109
41. Zaicev SY (2006) Supramolekularnye sistemy na granice razdela faz kak model membran i nanomaterialy (Supramolecular systems at interfaces as a model of membranes and nanomaterilas) Moscow state academy of veterinary and biotechnology, Moscow
42. Ivancev SS, Pavluchenko VN, Byrdina NA (1987) Elementary reactions of the emulsions polymerization of styrene with the localization of radical formation acts at the interface. J Polym Sci, Part A: Polym Chem 25:47–62
43. Voronov S et al (1996) Peroxidation of the interface of colloidal systems as new possibilities for design of compounds. Progr Colloid Polym Sci 101:189–193
44. Voronov S et al (2000) Polyperoxide surfactants for interface modification and compatibilization of polymer colloidal systems. I. Synthesis and properties of polyperoxide surfactants. J Appl Polym Sci 76:1217–1227
45. Taued K, Kosmella S (1993) Synthesis, characterization and application of surface active intiators. Polym Int 30:253–258
46. Stoffelbach F (2008) Use of a simple surface active initiator in controlled/living free-radical miniemulsion polymerization under AGET and ARGET ATRP conditions. Chem Comm. doi:10.1039/b809163c
47. Cheng CJ et al (2013) Facile synthesis of gemini surface active ATRP initiator and its use in soap-free AGET ATRP mini-emulsion polymerization. Chem Papers 67:336–341
48. Kohut A et al (2007) Macroinitiators on the basis of new peroxide surface active monomers. Chem Chem Technol 1:83–86
49. Zicmanis A et al (1997) Synthesis of new alkyl maleates ammonium derivatives and their uses in emulsion polymerization. Colloid Polym Sci 275:1–8

50. Abele S et al (1999) Cationic and zwitterionic polymerizable surfactants: quaternary ammonium dialkyl maleates. 1. Synthesis and characterization. Langmuir 15:1033–1044
51. Xu J, Li G, Zhou G, Yao F (2001) Synthesis and properties of novel cationic maleic diester polyerizable surfactants. Chin Chem Lett 12:523–526
52. Liangxian H et al (2008) Preparation and properties of a novel alkyl ethoxy carboxylate surfactant (CNKI). Speciality Petrochemicals 6:58
53. Yoshimura T, Koide Y, Shosenji H, Esumi K (2002) Preparation and surface active properties of telomere type anionic surfactant from maleic anhydride. J Surfactants Deterg 5:257–262
54. Rasika MS, Manohar RS (2006) Synthesis of amphoteric surfactants via esterification process. J Dispers Sci Technol 27:407–411
55. Yang SF et al (2005) St-Ba copolymer emulsions prepared by using novel cationic maleic dialkyl polimerizable emulsifier. Eur Polym J 41:2973–2979
56. Weihong L, Lai YC (2009) Novel polymerizable surface active monomers with both fluorine-containing groups and hydrophilic groups. US Patent 8071704 B2, 9 Apr 2009
57. Pich A et al (2005) Polymeric particles prepared with fluorinated surfmer. Polymer 46:1323–1330
58. Klimenkovsa I, Zhukovskaa I, Uzulinaa I, Zicmanis A (2003) Maleic diamide polymerizable surfactants. Applications in emulsion polymerization. C R Chim 6:1295–1304
59. Chen KM, Tsai CC (1988) Synthesis and surface active properties of maleic anhydride-polyethylene glycol-phthalic anhydride polymeric surfactants. J Am Oil Chem Soc 8:1346–1349
60. Vuitsyk LB (2009) Sintez monomeriv i iniciatoriv na osnovi mono- ta polisaharydiv (Synthesis of monomers and initiators based on mono- and polysaccharides). Dissertation, Lviv Polytechnic National University
61. Hevus O, Kohut A, Fleychuk R, Mitina N, Zaichenko O (2007) Colloid systems based on the basis of novel reactive surfmers. Macromolecular symposia, selected contributions from the 3rd international symposium on react 2007 254:117–121
62. Kohut AM, Hevus OI, Voronov SA (2004) Synthesis and properties of 4-(ω-methoxyoligodi methylsiloxanyl)butylmaleate; a new surfmer. J Appl Polym Sci 93:310–313
63. Borzenkov M, Hevus O (2013) Synthesis and properties of novel surface active monomers containing phosphate group. In: Abstracts of European polymer congress EPF-2013, Pisa, Italy, 16–21 June 2013
64. Buller K, Pearson D (1973) Organic Synthesis, vol 2. Mir, Moscow Russian Translation
65. Borzenkov MM (2012) Sintez i vlastuvosti poverhnevo-aktuvnyh monomeriv—pohidnyh hydroxy- ta aminocarbonovyh kislot (Synthesis and properties of surface active monomers based on derivatives of hydroxy and amino carboxylic acids). Dissertation, Lviv Polytechnic National University
66. Borzenkov MM, Hevus OI (2012) Novel peroxide containing maleate surface active monomers for obtaining reactive polymers. Macromol Symposia 315:60–65
67. Atta AM, Dyab AK, Allohedan HA (2013) A novel route to prepare highly surface activate nanogel particles based on nonaqueous emulsion polymerization. Polym Adv Technol 24:986–996
68. Cava MP et al (1974) N-phenylmaleimide. Org Synth 5:944
69. Huang CD, Tliba O (2005) G-protein-coupled receptor agonists differentially regulate basal or tumor necrosis factor-alpha-stimulated activation of interleukin-6 and RANTES in human airway smooth muscle cells. J Biomed Sc 12:763–776
70. Trivedi B (1982) Maleic Anhydride. Culberston, New York
71. Kim Y et al (2008) Efficient site-specific labeling of proteins via cysteins. Biocon Chem 19:786–791
72. Rich DH et al (1975) Alkylating derivatives of amino acids and peptides. Synthesis of N-maleoyl acids. J Med Chem 18:1004
73. Skrifvars M, Schmidt HW (1995) Synthesis of N-(2,5-Dicarboxyphenyl) maleimide. Synth Commun 25:1809–1815

74. Kozlowski A (2012) Compositions comprising conjugates and maleamic acid-terminated, water-soluble polymers. US patent 20120271000 A1, 25 Oct 2012
75. Ananda K et al (2008) Analysis of functionalization of methoxy-PEG as maleimide-PEG. Anal Biochem 374:231–242
76. Daniel HD et al (2005) Site-specific PEGylation of engineered cystein analogs of recombinant human granulocyte-macrophage colony stimulating factor. Bioconjug Chem 16:1291–1298
77. Roberts MJ, Bentley MD, Harris JM (2002) Chemistry for peptide and protein PEGylation. Adv Drug Deliv Rev 54:459–476
78. Lu Y et al (2008) Effect of PEGylation on the solution conformation of antibody fragments. J Pharm Sci 97:2062–2079
79. Felix FS et al (2011) In situ maleimide bridging of disulfides and a new approach to protein PEGylation. Bioconjug Chem 22:132–136
80. Prabhakaran M, Manjula BN, Acharya SA (2006) Molecular modeling studies of surface decoration of hemoglobin by maleimide PEG. Artif Cells Blood Substit Immobil Biotechnol 34:381–393
81. Accardo A et al (2011) Naposomes: a new class of peptide-derivatized, target-selective multimodal nanoparticles for imaging therapeutic applications. Ther Deliv 2:235–257
82. Liebher RB et al (2012) Maleimide activation of photon upconverting nanoparticles for bioconjugation. Nanotechnology 23. doi:10.1088/0957-4484/23/48/485103
83. Dispinar T, Sanyal R, Sanyal A (2007) A Diels–Alder/retro Diels–Alder strategy to synthesize polymers bearing maleimide-side chains. J Polym Sci, Part A: Polym Chem 45:4545–4551
84. Gandini A (2013) The furan/maleimide Diels–Alder reaction. A versatile click-unclick tool in macromolecular synthesis. Prog Polym Sci 38:1–29
85. Ganapathippan S, Zhou ZL (2011) Maleimide-containing latex dispersions. US patent, 7910649 B2, 22 Mar 2011
86. Tsotumo O et al (1994) Synthesis and polymerization of maleimides containing cholesteryl group. Polym J 26:1332–1344
87. Goutayer M et al (2010) Tumor targeting of fictionalized lipid nanoparticles: assessment by in vivo fluorescence imaging. J Pharm Biopharm 75:137–147
88. Cianga L, Yagci Y (2002) Synthesis and characterization of thiophene-substituted N-phenyl maleimide polymers by photoinduced radical polymerization. J Polym Sci, Part A: Polym Chem 40:995–1004
89. McElhanon J et al (2005) Thermally cleavable based on furan-meleimide Diels–Alder adducts. Langmuir 8:3259–3266
90. Thanamongkollit K et al (2012) Highly porous polymeric foam of maleimide-terminated poly(arylene ether sulfone) oligomers via high internal phase emulsions. Adv Sci Technol 77:165–171
91. Greene BW, Sheetz DP, Filler TD (1970) In situ polymerization of surface-active agents on latex particles. I. Preparation and characterization of styrene-butadiene latexes. J Colloid Interf Sci 32:90–95
92. Juang MS, Krieger IM (1976) Emulsifier-free emulsion polymerization with ionic comonomer. J Polym Sci, Part A: Polym Chem 14:2089–2107
93. Maliukova EB et al (1991) Emulsionnaya sopolimerizacia vinilovuh I dienovuh monomerov s poverhnostno-aktivnymi somonomerami (Emulsion copolymerization of vinyl and dienic monomers with surface active comonomers). High Mol Compd 33:1469–1475
94. Zaicev SY (2010) Supermolecularnye nanorazmernue sistemy na granice razdela faz. Koncepcyi i perspectivy dlia bionanotechnologiy (Supermolecular nanosystems at interface. Conceptions and opportunities for bionanotechnology). Lenand, Moscow
95. Zaicev SY (2009) Membrannie nanostructury na osnove biologiceski aktivnyh soedineniy dlia biotechnologii (Membrane nanostructures based on biological active compounds for biotechnology). Nanoreviews 4:46
96. Zaiceva LG, Ovchinnikova TV, Grinevich VA (2009) Import belkov v mitohondriah (Import of proteins in mitochondrion). Bioorg Chem 26:643–661

97. Shtilmann MI (2006) Polymery Medico-Biologiceskogo Znacenia (Polymers of Bio-Medical Application). Academbook, Moscow
98. Zaitsev SY, Baryshnikova EA, Veresschetin VP (1997) Polymerization of the 12-methacry-loyloxydodecanoic acid and a corresponding phospholipid in monolayers at the liquid-gas interfaces. Macromol Chem Macromol Symp 113:197
99. Ulman A (1991) An Introduction to Ultrathin Organic Films from Langmuir-Blodgett to Self-Assembly. Academic Press, Boston
100. Zaitsev SY, Moebius D (1994) Monolayers of Na, K-adenosine triphosphotase at the gas liquid interface. Thin Solid Films 244:890–894
101. Melehova EM, Kurochkin IN (1990) Teoreticeskoe rasmotrenie kineticeskih zakonomernos-tei processov vzaimodeistvia system vtoricnyh messehgerov pri aktivacyi kletki vneshnim himiceskim signalom (Theoretical basis of kinetics process of interaction of secondary mes-sengers during activation of cell by external chemical signal). Mol Biol 24:1261
102. Kohut A, Hevus O, Voronov S (2000) Copolymers on the basis of ω-aminoalkyl acrylates and quaternary ammonium salts. In: Abstracts of Polish–Ukrainian conference on polymers of special application, Radom, Poland
103. Black WA et al (1969) The synthesis of polymerizable vinyl sugars. Makromol Chem 122:244
104. Narain R, Armes S (2003) Synthesis and aqueous solutions properties of novel sugar meth-acrylate based homopolymers and block copolymers. Biomacromolecules 4:1746–1758
105. Borzenkov M, Hevus O (2014) Synthesis of novel surface active methacrylate monomers based on ε-caprolactone. Chem Chem Technol 8:141–146
106. Klee EJ, Lehmann U (2010) Novel 2-(ω-phosphonooxy-2-oxaalkyl)acrylate monomers for self-etching self-priming one part adhesive. Beilstein J Org Chem 6:766–772
107. Shalaby S, Ikada Y, Langer R (1993) Polymers of biological and biomedical significance. ACS Pub 540:191
108. Cho HG (2010) Preparation and characterization of novel acrylic monomers. J Appl Polym Sci 116:736–742
109. Vries AR (2006) Novel monomer for hydrophilic acrylic copolymers and their novel proper-ties. Dissertation, University of Stanford, USA
110. Li W, Matjaszewski K (2011) Cationic surface-active monomers as reactive surfactants for AGET Emulsion ATRP of n-butyl methacrylate. Macromolecules 44:5578
111. Hamid MS, Sherington DC (1987) Novel quaternary ammonium amphiphilyc (meth) acrylates: 2. Thermally and photochemically initiated polymerization. Polymer 28:332–339
112. Luo N et al (2002) Synthesis of a novel methacrylic monomer iniferter and its application in surface photografting on crosslinked polymer substrates. J Polm Sci. Part A 40:1885
113. Pekel N et al (2004) Synthesis and characterization of poly(N-vinylimidazole-co-acryloni-trile) and determination of monomers reactivity ratios. Macromol Chem Physic 205:1039
114. Thomas R et al (1997) Preparation and surface properties of acrylic polymers containing fluorinated monomers. Macromolecules 30:2883–2890
115. Ishihara K et al (2006) Water structure and improved mechanical properties of phospholipid pol-ymer hydrogel with phosphorylcholine centered intermolecular cross-linker. Polymer 47:1390
116. Ishihara K et al (2006) UCST-type cononosolvency behavior of poly (2-methacryloxyethyl phosphorylcholine) in the mixture of water and ethanol. Polym J 40:479–483
117. Senhaj O et al (2004) Synthesis and characterization of new methacrylic phosphonated sur-face active monomer. Macromol Chem Phys 205:1039
118. Hevus I, Pikh Z (2007) Novel surfactants for creating reactive polymers. Macromol Symposia 1:103–108
119. Choi SW (2013) Bis(vinylcyclopropane) and bis(methacrylate) monomers with cholesteryl group for dental composites. e-Polymers 5:820–831
120. He J et al (2011) Synthesis of methacrylate monomers with antibacterial effects against *S Mutans*. Macromolecules 16:9755–9763
121. Al-Sabagh AM (2012) Novel polymerizable nonionic surfactants (surfmers) corporate with alkenylsuccinic anhydride: synthesis, surface, and thermodynamic properties. J Disp Sci Tech 33:1458–1469

122. Sakai K et al (2009) Polymerizable anionic gemeni surfactants: physicochemical properties in aqueous solution and polymerization behavior. J Oleo Sci 58:403–413
123. Ma L et al (2014) Synthesis and micellar behaviors of an anionic polymerizable surfactant. J Chin Chem Soc. doi:10.1002/jccs.201300372
124. Ilan AH (1992) Low-temperature transmission electron microscopy and differential scanning calorimetry characterization of latexes stabilized with surface active block oligomers. Polymer 33:2043–2050
125. Busci A et al (1998) Monodisperse polysterene latex particles functionalized by the macromonomer technique. Macromolecules 31:581–620
126. Chao D, Itsuno S, Ito K (1991) Poly(ethylene oxide) macromonomers. Synthesis and polymerization of macromonomers carrying styryl end groups with enhanced hydrophobicity. Polym J 23:1045–1052
127. Ito K, Tanaka K, Tanaka H (1991) Poly(ethylene oxide) macromonomers. Micellar polymerization in water. Macromolecules 24:2348–2354
128. Soula O et al (1993) Styrenic surfmer in emulsion copolymerization of acrylic monomers. Copolymerization and film properties. J Polym Sci Part A Polym Chem Ed 37:4202–4217
129. Narain R, Jhury D, Wulff G (2002) Synthesis and characterization of polymers on 4-vinyl-phenylglucitiol. Eur Polym J 38:273
130. Klein J, Herzog D, Hajibegli A (1985) Polyvinylsaccharides. Synthesis and characterization of new polyvinylsaccarides of the urea type. Makromol Chem Rapid Commun 6:675
131. Borzenkov M et al (2012) Synthesis and polymerizable properties of novel cationic surface active monomers based on derivatives of ω-bromo and ω-amino carboxylic acids. In: Ukrainian–Polish conference on polymers of special applications, Radom, 24–27 Sept 2012
132. Nagasaki Y, Takahashi T, Tsuruta T (1990) Synthesis of novel functional styrene monomers having trimethylsilyl and hydroxyalkyl groups by the reaction between 4-vinylbenzyllithium derivatives and oxiranes. Die Makromolekulare Chemie 191:2297
133. Ocampo-Fernandez M et al (2009) Synthesis and characterization of diethyl-p-vinylbenzyl phosphonate monomer: precursor for ion exchange polymers for fuel cells. Superficies y Vacio 22:6–10
134. Wu H, Kawaguchi S, Ito K (2004) Synthesis and polymerization of tale-type polymerizable surfactants and hydrophobic counter-anion induced association of polyelectrolytes. Coll and Polym Sci 282:1365–1373

Chapter 2
Colloidal Properties of Surface Active Monomers

2.1 Colloidal Properties of Surfactants

A surfactants ("surface-active agents") are defined as a materials that can greatly reduce the surface tension of water when used in appointed concentrations. This concentration is known as critical micelle concentration (CMC) determined as the concentration of surfactants above which micelles form and all additional surfactants added to the system go to micelles [1]. Surfactants are amphiphilic compounds containing both hydrophobic groups and hydrophilic groups [2]. Therefore, they contain oil-soluble and water-soluble components. The typical changing of values of surface tension of water when adding a surfactant is shown on Scheme 2.1.

While reaching the CMC, the values of surface tension change strongly with the concentration of the surfactant [1]. After reaching the CMC, the surface tension is almost constant or changes with a lower slope. At the concentrations above CMC, the micelles, which are determined as an aggregate of surfactants, are formed [3]. From the bases of colloidal chemistry, it is known that the classical micelle in aqueous solutions consists of two main parts, namely the hydrophilic "head" regions in contact with solvent and hydrophilic tails in the micelle center [4]. The typical structure of micelle is shown on Scheme 2.2.

With the increase of micelle size, the micelle shape can change from spherical to rod-like or to dimensional disk-like aggregates. The self-assembly of surfactants depends on the length of alkyl chain, the nature of hydrophilic "head," the salt concentration, pH, and temperature [5].

Specific amphiphilic molecules, such as lipids, are capable to form closed bilayer assemblies in aqueous solution known as vesicles [6]. Special attention is paid to these systems due to their ability to mimic biological cell membranes [7]. Vesicles are larger than micelles, which have a smaller surface curvature and higher degree of organization [6]. The simplest image of vesicle is displayed on Scheme 2.3.

© The Author(s) 2014
M. Borzenkov and O. Hevus, *Surface Active Monomers*,
SpringerBriefs in Materials, DOI: 10.1007/978-3-319-08446-6_2

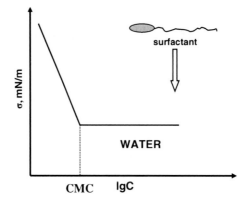

Scheme 2.1.1 Typical surface tension isotherm showing the decrease of surface tension when surfactant is added. The inflection point corresponds to CMC

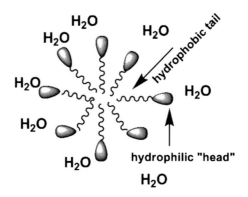

Scheme 2.1.2 The structure of typical micelle in aqueous solution

The above-described bases of surfactants colloidal properties are *background* of colloidal properties of surface-active monomers. Therefore, the next subchapter concentrates on colloidal behavior of surfmers.

2.2 Fundamentals of Colloidal Chemistry of Surface-Active Monomers

It was already told in introduction that surface-active monomers during the preparation of emulsion of monomers in water are located predominantly on the monomer droplet–water interface, thus acting as surfactants stabilizing the emulsion. Colloidal properties of surface-active monomers like in case of traditional surfactants depend on length and origin of lipophilic and hydrophilic fragments.

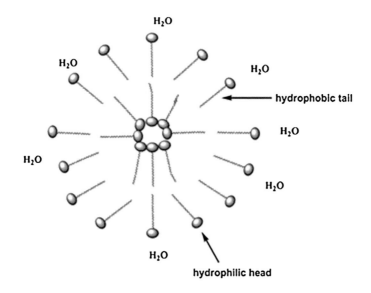

Scheme 2.3 The scheme of a vesicle formed in aqueous solution

   Like typical surfactants, the surface-active monomers most commonly classified according to polar "head" group. A non-ionic surfmers have no charge groups
in their "head." If the charge on the "head" is negative, the surfmers are considered
as anionic, and if the charge on the "head" is positive, the surfmers are called cationic. In case surfmer contains a "head" with two oppositely charged groups, it is
called zwitterionic. This classification is displayed on the Scheme 2.4.
   Some typical for surfmers ionic groups are shown on the Scheme 2.5.
   The anionic hydrophilic group can influence on a range of parameters: the elec-
trostatic stabilization, the sensitivity to pH, and electrolyte condition. Zwitterionic
surfmers can be anionic and cationic or both depending on the structure and
medium conditions.
   As it was told in introduction, polymerizable part in the molecule of surfmer
could be located either in hydrophilic or hydrophobic part or between these two parts.
   As opposite to typical monomers, surface-active monomers due to their surface-active properties are characterized by the micelle formation and the adsorption at interfaces [8]. Surfmers are capable to form both true and micellar solutions
in water [9]. Also, the surface-active monomers which are structural analogous
of phospholipids can form structures resembling biological membranes in solution (vesicles and liposomes) [10] and at the interface (monolayers and polylay-
ers) [10]. Surface-active monomers provide an opportunity for developing hybrid
nanosized reaction and templating media with constrained geometries [6].
   CMC of surfmers is an essential characteristic and a key point for further application of these compounds. Actually, it is the concentration where the surfmer acts
as micelle. Micellization is a strongly cooperative self-association process accru-
ing at a narrow concentration of surfmer [11]. Surface tension measurements are

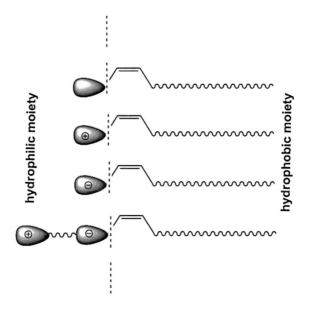

Scheme 2.4 Classification of surfmers according to polarity: non-ionic, cationic, anionic, and zwitterionic

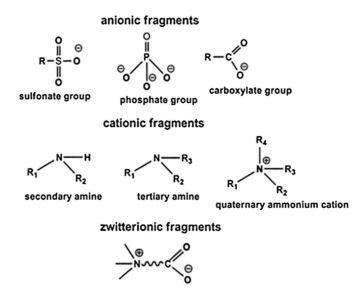

Scheme 2.5 Some typical ionic groups incorporated in structure of surfmers

generally used for CMC determination. Nevertheless, there are other physical properties that can be used to monitor micelle formation and CMC determination. For example, the rate of increase in osmotic pressure falls into a plateu [11].

A sharp increase in turbidity is also observed by light-scattering techniques [11]. In conductance measurements, a marked decrease in the slope is observed after crossing CMC indicating that there are much less mobile charged units than expected from the individual surfactants molecules [11]. The so-called hydrophobic effect is considered as a main driving force in self-association that is an entropic driven process [3, 11]. The self-assembly of surfmers like in case of traditional surfactants depends on a range of factors such as length of hydrophobic tail, surfmer concentration, nature of hydrophilic moiety, pH, and temperature. The presence of long hydrophobic chain promotes the poor solubility of surface-active monomers. Therefore, the corresponding monomers form micelles under low concentrations. The introducing of hydrophilic groups of various nature and hydrophobic chains of different length gives an opportunity to vary the surface-active properties of synthesized surfmers in wide range. Since the first publications devoted to colloidal properties of surfmers were appeared, numerous of corresponding papers have been published. For the convenience, the following subchapters focus more on properties and polymerization of micelles, vesicles, mesophases or lyotropic liquid crystals, and microemulsions.

2.3   Properties and Polymerization of Micelles, Vesicles, Mesophases or Lyotropic Liquid Crystals, and Microemulsions

2.3.1   Micelles

One of the earliest publications devoted to micelle polymerization was made by Larrabee and Sprague [12]. The polymerization was only observed at concentration of surfmer above the CMC proving that micelle formation is essential condition of polymerization. This is a typical phenomenon observed with all surface-active monomers and is explained by "condensation effect of monomer" [13], which makes an accelerated propagation step [6]. Polymerization of surfmers in micelles and other self-assembled phases has been studied for at least 30 years. The polymerization process is strongly influenced by the structure and properties of the micelles. The term "polymerized micelle" was discussed in publications of Sherrington et al. [14–16]. He proposed that during the polymerization process, the formation of "polysoap," an oligomeric species that exhibits micellar-like physical properties. The schematic representation of "polymerized micelle" and "polysoap" is shown on Scheme 2.6.

The monomer reactivity and location o polymerizable appreciably impact on the nature of polymerizable species [17]. During the last decade, it has observed a substantial advance in understanding both the structure and dynamics of polymerizable surfmer micelles. In the review published in 2012, the new insights yielded primarily by small-angle neutron scattering using high-flux sources were highlighted [18]. This technique provides further prospects for realizing and controlling topochemical polymerization in micellar systems.

(a)   **(b)**

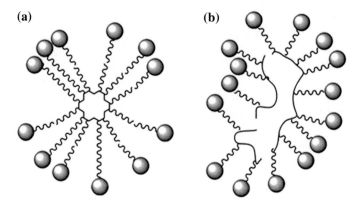

Scheme 2.6 Schematic representation of "polymerized micelle" (**a**) and "polysoap" (**b**)

The physicochemical properties in aqueous solution of synthesized anionic gemini surfmer containing two anionic monomeric parts linked with an ethylene spacer and polymerizable methacryloxy groups covalently bound to the terminal of the hydrocarbon chains were studied [19]. In the region of low added electrolyte concentrations, the synthesized surfmer spontaneously formed spherical micelles in aqueous solution, which was confirmed with the Corrin-Harkins analysis (CMC vs. total counterion concentration) and cryogenic transmission electron microscopy. Al-Sabagh et al. [20] reported about the synthesis of novel surfmers with terminated terminal acrylate group on the hydrophilic moiety. In this work, the surface and thermodynamic parameters of the prepared surfmers were determined at 25 °C including surface tension and effectiveness maximum surface excess, and minimum surface area Also, the standard free energy of micellization and adsorption were recorded. Micellization and surface-active properties of hydrocarbon and fluorocarbon surfmers were reported in a paper published in Langmuir [21]. The interaction between synthesized surfmers in aqueous micellar state and solubilization capacity was reported. The CMC, fractional charge per micelle, and standard free energy change of micellization were determined for polymerizable sodium itaconate monoesters in a paper published in 2013 [22]. The effect of hydrophobic chain length of synthesized surfmers on micellization parameters was reported. In another paper published in 2013 in Journal of Surfactants and Detergents, micellization and adsorption of new reactive surfmers based on modified nonyl phenol ethoxylates were described [23]. Bunio and Chlebicki [24] characterized sorbic acid amphiphilic polymerizable derivatives. Interfacial activity and micellar properties of synthesized compounds were investigated.

Suresh and Bartsch [25] performed the evaluation of a newly developed anionic surfmer, sulfonated 3-pentadecyl phenyl acrylate, in the emulsion polymerization of styrene and its effect on the polymer properties. The obtained results were compared with the commercially available non-reactive anionic surfactant sodium lauryl sulfate. The corresponding surfmer has a low critical micellar concentration value of 40.11 mg/L in comparison with 2,400 mg/L for sodium dodecyl sulfate.

Zaragoza-Contreros et al. [26] reported about anilinium dodecylsulfate surfmer prepared from aniline and sodium dodecylsulfate for synthesis of polystyrene/polyaniline core-shell composites. The critical micellar concentration of the salt was determined using electrical conductimetry, which detected that the change of countercation, sodium by anilinium, reduced the CMC with respect to the conventional counterpart, sodium dodecylsulfate. In the paper published in 2012, mixed micelles composed of alcohol and hexadecyl trimethyl allylammonium chloride were constructed and their properties were studied [27]. An interesting result is reported in publication of Ohkubo et al. [28]. The authors synthesized and characterized the cationic gemini methacrylate surfmers. The equilibrium properties of surfmers in water were investigated by means of surface tension, and polymerization of resulted micelles was performed. The highly dispersed state of molecular assembly of gemini surfmer was considered as excellent property to prepare uniform polymer micelle without any flocculation of micelles. In the paper published in 2013 in Journal of Dispersion Science and Technology, the dynamics of surface activity and a range of parameters such as surface tension at the CMC, adsorption efficiency, and Gibbs free energy of the micellization were evaluated for novel cationic imidazolium surfmers [29]. The maximum surface excess concentration and minimum surface area/molecule at the air–water interface were also estimated. The micellar behaviors of surfmers of acrylamide type, sodium 2-acrylamido-tetradecane sulfonate and sodium 2-acrylamido-dodecane sulfonate, were studied [30]. It was found that the effects of the length of the hydrophobic hydrocarbon chain and the addition of electrolyte on the micellar behaviors for the anionic synthesized anionic surfmers of acrylamide type are similar to typical anionic surfactants. In the other paper, the micellization behavior of homopolymer of (2-acrylamido) ethyl tetradecyl dimethylammonium bromide was investigated [31]. In the paper published in 2012 in Journal of Colloid and Interface Science, an empirical model for the concentrations of monomeric and micellized surfactants as a consistent approach for the quantitative analysis of obtained data was presented [32]. The reported concentration model provided an objective definition of the CMC and yielded precise and well-defined values of physical parameters. Benbayer et al. [33] reported about characterization of novel hybrid hydrocarbon/fluorocarbon ammonium-type surfmers. The synthesized surfmers exhibited very low surface tension as well as low critical micellar concentrations. Obtained results indicated that the acrylic function has a pronounced effect on increasing the hydrophobic micelle character. In the paper published by Zhang et al. [34] in 2013, the comparison of a properties were made for pressure adhesives generated via emulsion polymerization using both conventional and polymerizable surfactants.

The surface activity of reported maleic surfmers [35] with hydrophobic alkylic, fluoroalkilic, and olygomethylsiloxanic could be managed by the nature of hydrophobic blocks. It was found the surface activity decreased in the following range fluoroalkilic > olygomethylsiloxanic > alkylic chain. The synthesized nonionic and ionic monomers [36] based on derivatives of 4-hydroxybutyric acid and 6-hydroxyhexanoic acid exhibited significant surface activity, and introducing of hydrophilic groups of various nature and hydrophobic chains of different length gives an opportunity to vary the surface-active properties of synthesized surfmers in wide range. Also, the synthesized recently saccharide containing monomers [37] are typical surfactants, since they reduce the surface tension on aqueous solution–air interface. As an example, the typical surface tension isotherms of some of above-mentioned surface are shown on Figs. 2.1, 2.2, and 2.3.

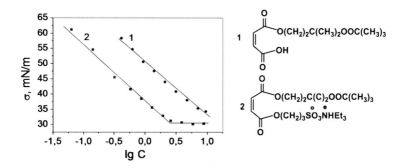

Fig. 2.1 Surface tension isotherms of synthesized maleate surfmers with containing di-tertperoxide group

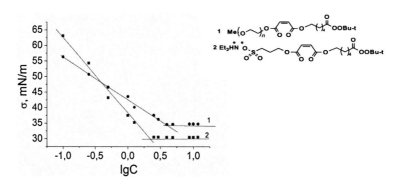

Fig. 2.2 Surface tension isotherms of surfmers containing peroxide groups synthesized from ε-caprolactone

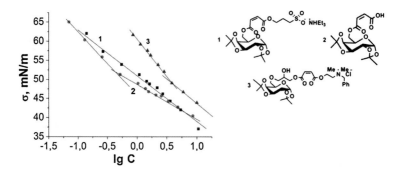

Fig. 2.3 Surface tension monomers of synthesized maleate saccharide containing monomers

Unusual surface tension isotherms of saccharide containing surfmers could be explained by the capability of diisopropylidengalactoside fragment to form associates with water [38]. This changes the orientation of corresponding compounds at interface.

2.3.2 Vesicles and Bilayers

Synthetic vesicles unlike naturally occurring systems tend to revert back to the lamellar phase by vesicle fusion or they precipitate out from an aqueous dispersion [39]. One of the best strategies to overcome this problem is to lock in these structures by the employment of surfmers [40, 41]. Polymerizable vesicles are formed by the functionalization of vesicle-forming surfactant with polymerizable groups. The organization and aggregation of the monomers and their dynamics in the vesicular phase impact on polymerization process and the structure of resulted polymers. Vesicles and liposomes are able to solubilize hydrophobic substances in the interior of their surfactant bilayer. Using hydrophobic monomers, subsequent polymerization leads to the formation of polymer chains entrapped in the hydrophobic part of the membrane. The schematic structure of a vesicle formed by surfmer is shown on Scheme 2.7.

The description of polymerizable vesicles was firstly reported in a publication of Regen et al. [42]. The enhanced stability of resulted polymerized vesicles was additionally confirmed by the unchanged absorbance during the addition of ethanol. The unique character of the bilayer vesicles was used to synthesize novel polymer architectures not available by conventional methods [6]. This statement was confirmed by O'Brien et al. [43] while using novel two-tailed heterobifunctional

Scheme 2.7 Schematic structure of a vesicle formed by surfmer

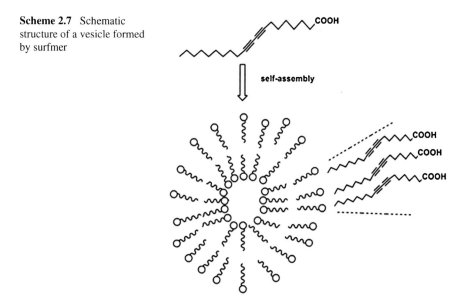

Scheme 2.8 Locations of polymerizable groups in the structure of reactive lipids

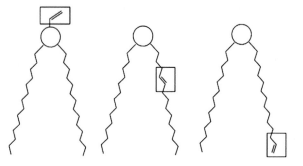

lipid, containing a diene and a dienoyl group in a single chain. The difference in polarity of the local environment of each reactive group within the vesicle made it possible to perform either simultaneous or selective polymerization, depending on the mode of initiation. The employing of mixtures of mono- and bis-substituted monomers allows the cross-link density of the poly(lipid) structure to be varied accordingly and provides a convenient way of modifying the physical properties of the final polymer [6]. The schematic presentation of the different locations of polymerizable groups in the structure of reactive lipids is shown on Scheme 2.8.

Jung et al. [44] showed that styrene and divinyl benzene could be successfully copolymerized in a bilayer matrix composed of single- or double-chained quaternary ammonium surfmer bearing one or two terminal styrene groups. It was found that unilamellar vesicles were formed with monofunctional surfmer, while the bisfunctional surfmer did not form vesicles itself, but could be incorporated into a matrix of monofunctional surfmer [6, 44]. The cross-linking activity of the bisfunctional surfmer enhanced the stability and produced rippled bilayer morphology [45].

Another interesting and prospective approach includes the utilization of vesicles with the polymerizable group as counterion. One unique feature of using a polymerizable counterion is the possibility of generating a coated vesicle or liposome in a net, in which the polymer network acts as a membrane that is not covalently linked but is electrostatically encasing the bilayers; the components of the lipid bilayer therefore retain their monomeric state [39]. Regen et al. [46] described surfmer with a potentially cross-linkable diallylammonium group as a counterion. One potential drawback with the Regen systems is that the diallylammonium counterions are known to undergo cyclopolymerization to produce linear rather than cross-linked systems and the extent of cross-linking in vesicles might have been limited. In the paper published in Journal of Polymer Science in 2004, counterion surfmers, dicetyldimethylammonium 4-vinyl benzoate, and dicetyldimethylammonium 3,5-divinyl benzoate were synthesized and, as expected, these surfmers formed both homo and mixed vesicles which were readily polymerized with a suitable radical photo-initiator [39].

To prepare vesicles with polymerizable bilayers lipids with polymerizable moieties usually needs to be synthesized, and this often involves multistep reactions. Therefore, Lee et al. [47] proposed an alternative, simpler approach based on a commercially available, single-tailed surfactant, 10-undecenoic acid, a fatty acid with a terminal double-bond. It was shown that 10-undecenoic acid can also be induced to form vesicles by adjusting the pH: vesicles form at intermediate pH (6–8), whereas at higher pH, the vesicles are transformed into micelles. The presence of 10-undecenoic acid vesicles in the pH 6–8 range was confirmed using small-angle neutron scattering and cryotransmission electron microscopy. Subsequent thermal polymerization of 10-undecenoic acid bilayers was carried out using 2,2-dimethoxy-2-phenylacetophenone as initiator. Kaler et al. [48] synthesized cationic methacryloyloxyundecyl trimethylammonium bromide and anionic sodium 4-(ω-methacryloyloxyundecyl)oxy benzene sulfonate and showed that the microstructures formed by mixtures of these surfmers in aqueous solution include stable vesicles, the structure of which can be fixed by polymerization. Another interesting types of surfmers which are capable to form vesicles were introduced in a publication of Bordes et al. [49] published in Langmuir in 2007. In this work, a new family of polymerizable surfactants was synthesized starting from a 1:1 mixture of alkylcarboxylic acids (C_{10}–C_{16}) and norbornene methyleneamine. Light-scattering measurements and electron microscopy observations confirmed the spontaneous formation of stable vesicles (90 nm $< d <$ 370 nm). Also, NMR experiments showed the enclosing of the norbornene part inside the vesicle membrane.

2.3.3 Lyotropic Liquid Crystals

Lyotropic Liquid Crystals (LLC) assemblies have garnered widespread attention in disparate areas of chemistry. Condensed high-curvature LLC or mesophases, with well-ordered periodic nanodomains offer grate potential as templates for mesoporous inorganic materials, as media for biophysical studies of transmembrane proteins ("cubic lipidic phases"), and as therapeutic nucleic acid delivery vehicles [6]. LLCs form by the concentration-dependent supramolecular self-organization of amphiphilic molecules in water into soft materials having distinct hydrophilic and hydrophobic nanoscale domains with long-range periodic order. Moreover, the organized polar and non-polar domains in lyotropic liquid crystalline phases provide an excellent opportunity to produce polymers with geometries and functionalities which cannot be achieved through traditional bulk or solution polymerization. One of the ways that is used for generation of nanostructured material to LLC media is utilization of surfmers to form structured materials on a nanometer scale. The organization of surfmers in LLC phases can have a large influence on the polymerization behavior by changing the local concentration of reactive groups and restricting the diffusion of propagating monomers and polymers [50]. The hydrophilic and hydrophobic domains of LLC can allow confinement of reactants within well-defined dimensions. LLC monomer can assembled into lamellar, hexagonal, and cubic structures according to the molecular structure, type, and content of solvent and temperature. The importance of LLC order during polymerization of monomeric lipids is highlighted in the publications of O'Brain et al. [43, 51] which demonstrate significant alteration of physical properties when lipids are polymerized in ordered LLC phases. The channel dimensions in the inverse hexagonal structure can be tailored by modifying the length of the hydrocarbon chain of surfmer [50]. Varying the position of the polymerizable group, the tail length, and the counterion of the head group, feature size may be tailored to allow tuning off the properties of resulted materials [50]. The development of functional materials with nanometer-scale architectures and the effect of these architectures on their chemical and physical properties are of great interest in materials design. The studies devoted to formation and polymerizations of LLC carried out in 1980th–1990th are well reported in works of O'Brien et al. [43], McGrath KM and Drummond [52], and McGrath [53]. The applications of polymerized LLC assemblies were discussed in a paper published in 2001 [54].

The biocontinuous cubic lyotropic liquid crystal networks formed by synthesized polymerizable gemini ammonium surfactants is reported in a paper published in 2010 [55]. Another types and application of novel gemini surfmers capable for forming the lyotropic liquid crystal networks is described in US patent published in 2013 [56]. The corresponding anionic surfmers containing at least seven carbon atoms may be used to prepare triply periodic multiply continuous lyotropic phase and polymers thereof that substantially retain triply periodic multiply continuous lyotropic phase structure. The application of ammonium-type gemini surfmers applied for the formation of LLC crystal network was also reported in another US patent published in 2012 [57]. In this patent, a new Q_I-phase gemini LLC monomer system has been developed. Homologs of this gemini ammonium-based monomer system exhibited Q_I phases that could be cross-linked with retention of the structure. The use of methacrylate surfmer, dodecyldimethylammonium ethyl methacrylate, for fabrication polymeric carbon nanotube–liquid crystal composites was reported by Kwon et al. [58]. The bare LC of corresponding surfmer and the dispersions showed columnar hexagonal phases. The nanotubes were well incorporated in the hexagonal LC phase where they induced a swelling of the structure. The advances in the design of polymerizable LLC assemblies are discussed in number of publications [59–62].

2.3.4 Microemulsions

Miniemulsions are a special class of emulsions that are stabilized against coalescence (by a surfactant) and Ostwald ripening (by an osmotic pressure agent) [63]. A major difference between emulsions and microemulsions comes from the amount of surfactant needed to stabilize the systems. Microemulsions exhibit unique microenvironments for performing chemistry, and therefore, there has been a lot of interest devoted to the use of these systems as host media for polymerization reactions [6]. The basic feature of performing polymerization in microemulsion is that in these systems, nucleation can take place directly inside very small monomer droplets. The miniemulsions are produced by high-energy homogenization and usually yield stable and narrowly distributed droplets with a size ranging from 50 to 500 nm. The first surveys in this field were carried out in the early 1980s by Stoffer and Thomas [64, 65]. In the pioneering studies, the utilization of non-polymerizable surfactants as stabiliziers, such as sodium dodecyl sulfate, often led to phase separation. Later, it was that found that incorporation of surfmers instead of traditional surfactant can solve the range of problems during miniemulsion polymerization [66]. The microemulsion polymerization in the presence of surfmers is discussed in the next chapter.

For conclusion, it should be said that surface-active properties of surfmers, namely the capability to form micelles and vesicles, and combination of the length of hydrophobic chain and a nature of hydrophilic part open a large opportunities for performing various polymerization techniques. The next chapter is devoted to polymerizable behavior of these compounds.

References

1. Ruckenstein E, Nagarajan R (1975) Critical micelle concentration. A transition point for micellar size distribution. J Phys Chem 79:2622–2626
2. Scott MJ, Malcolm N (2000) The biodegradation of surfactants in the environment. Biochimica et Biophysica Acta (BBA). Biomembranes 1508:235–251
3. Tranford C (1980) The hydrophobic effect. The formation of micelles and biological membranes. Wiley, New York
4. Rosen MJ (1989) Surfactants and interfacial phenomena. Wiley, New York
5. Malmsten M (2002) Surfactants and polymers in drug delivery. Taylor & Francis, New York
6. Summers M, Eastoe J (2003) Applications of polymerizable surfactants. Adv Colloid Interface Sci 100–102:137–152
7. Lin Q, London E (2014) Preparation of artificial plasma membrane mimicking vesicles with lipid asymmetry. PLoS ONE 9(1). doi:10.1371/journal.pone.008790
8. Holmberg K (1992) Polymerizable surfactants. Prog Org Coat 20:235–241
9. Egorov VV, Zubov VP (1987) Radical polymerization in the associated species of ionogenic surface active monomers in water. Russ Chem Rev 56:2076–2097 (Translated from Uspekhi Khimii)
10. Zaicev SY (2010) Supermolecularnye nanorazmernue sistemy na granice razdela faz. Koncepcyi i perspectivy dlia bionanotechnologiy (Supermolecular nanosystems at interface. Conceptions and opportunities for bionanotechnology). Lenand, Moscow
11. Santos S (2013) Amphiphilic molecules in drug delivery systems. In: Coelho J (ed) Drug delivery systems: advanced technologies potentially applicable is personalized treatment. doi:10.1007/978-94-007-6010-3_2
12. Larabee CE, Sprague ED (1979) Radiation-induced polymerization of sodium 10-undecenoate in aqueous micelle solutions. J Polym Sci Polym Let Ed 17:749–751
13. Aida T, Tajima K (2000) Controlled polymerization with constrained geometries. Chem Commun 24:2399–2412
14. Sherington DC, Hamid SM (1987) Novel quaternary ammonium amphiphilic (meth) acrylates: 1. Synthesis, melting and interfacial behavior. Polymer 28:325–331
15. Joynes D, Sherington DC (1996) Novel polymerizable mono- and divalent quaternary ammonium cationic surfactants: 1. Synthesis, structural characterization and homopolymerization. Polymer 37:1453–1462
16. Sherington DC, Joynes D (1997) Novel polymerizable mono- and divalent quaternary ammonium cationic surfactants: 2. Surface active properties and use in emulsion polymerization. Polymer 38:1427–1438

17. Dais P et al (1993) Positional effects of the methacrylate group on polymerization and micro-structure of micelle-forming quaternary ammonium salts studied by NMR spectroscopy. Macromol Chem 194:445–450
18. Fitzgerald PA, War GG (2012) Structure of polymerizable surfactant micelles: insights from neutron scattering. Adv Colloid Interface Sci 179–182:14–21
19. Sakai K et al (2009) Polymerizable anionic gemeni surfactants: physicochemical properties in aqueous solution and polymerization behavior. J Oleo Sci 58:403–413
20. Al-Sabagh AM et al (2012) Novel polymerizable nonionic surfactants (surfmers) corporate with alkenylsuccinic anhydride: synthesis, surface, and thermodynamic properties. J Disp Sci Tech 33:1458–1469
21. Stähler K et al (1998) Novel hydrocarbon and fluorocarbon polymerizable surfactants: synthesis, characterization and mixing behavior
22. Prabha DR, Santhaanalakshmi J, Arun Prasath R (2013) Analysis of micellar behavior of a synthesized sodium itaconate monoesters with various hydrophobic chain lengths in aqueous media. Res J Chem Sci 12:43–49
23. Atta A, Dyab A, Al-Lohedan H (2013) Micellisation and adsorption behaviors of new reactive polymerizable surfactants based on modified nonyl phenol ethoxylates. J Surf Det 16:343
24. Bunio P, Chlebicki J (2012) Novel sorbic-type quaternary ammonium single-chain and gemini polymerizable surfactants: synthesis, interfacial properties and anti-electrostatic activity. Colloids Surf A 413:119–124
25. Suresh IK, Bartsch E (2013) Effect of sulfonated 3-pentadecyl phenyl acrylate as surfmer in the emulsion polymerization of styrene: synthesis and polymer properties. Colloid Polym Sci 291:1843–1853
26. Zaragoza-Contreros EA et al (2012) Synthesis of core–shell composites using an inverse surfmer. J Colloid Interface Sci 377:231–236
27. Liu JX et al (2012) Polymerization of micro-block associative polymer with alcohol-surfmer mixed micellar method and their rheological properties. Acta Phys Chim Sin 28:1757–1763
28. Ohkubo T et al (2006) Nano-sized polymer micelle synthesized from cationic gemini surfmer. NSTI-Nanotech 1:64–67
29. Kaur C et al (2013) Synthesis and evaluation of surface active properties of esters-based cationic imidazolium monomeric surfactants. J Dispersion Sci Technol 34:1488–1495
30. Gao B, Yu Y, Jiang L (2007) Studies on micellar behavior of anionic and surface-active monomers with acrylamide type in aqueous solution. Colloid Surf A 293:210–216
31. Liu K, Li L (2008) Preparation and unimolecular micellization of behavior of homopolymer of surface active monomer AMC14AB. Chin J Chem Phys 21:469–475
32. Al-Suofi W, Pineiro L, Novo M (2012) A model for monomer and micellar concentration in surfactant solutions. Application and conductivity, NMR, diffusion and surface tension data. J Colloid Interface Sci. doi:10.1016/j.jcis.2011.12.037
33. Benbayer C et al (2013) Investigation of structure-surface properties relationship of semi-fluorinated polymerizable cationic surfactants. J Colloid Interface Sci 408:125–131
34. Zhang J et al (2013) Surface enrichment by conventional polymerizable sulfated nonylphenol ethoxylate emulsifiers in water based pressure-sensitive adhesive. Ind Eng Chem Res 52:8616–8621
35. Hevus O et al (2007) Colloidal systems on the basis of novel reactive surfmers. Macromol Symp 254:117–121
36. Borzenkov M, Hevus O (2012) Novel peroxide containing maleate surface active monomers for obtaining reactive polymers. Macromol Symp 315:60–65
37. Vuitsyk LB (2009) Sintez monomeriv i iniciatoriv na osnovi mono-ta polisaharydiv (Synthesis of monomers and initiators based on mono- and polysaccharides). Dissertation, Lviv Polytechnic National University
38. Zaikov G (2005) Chemistry of polysaccharides. Taylor & Francis Group, New York
39. Paul GK, Indi SS, Ramakrishnan S (2004) Synthesis and vesicular polymerization of novel counter-ion polymerizable/crosslinkable surfactants. J Polym Sci: Part A: Polym Chem 42:5271–5283

40. Paleos CM (1992) In Paleos CM (ed) Polymerization in organized media: Gordon Breach Science Publishers, Philadelphia
41. Im JY et al (2002) Surface modified porous polymeric membrane using vesicles. Bull Korean Chem Soc 232:1616–1622
42. Regen SL, Czeh D, Singh A (1980) Polymerized vesicles. J Am Chem Soc 102:6638–6640
43. O'Brien DF, Sisson TM, Srisiri W (1998) Novel polymer architectures via the selective polymerization of lyotropic liquid crystals of heterobifunctional amphiphiles. J Am Chem Soc 120:2322–2329
44. Jung M et al (2000) Polymerization in polymerizable vesicle bilayer membrane. Langmuir 16:4185–4195
45. O'Brien DF, Liu S (1999) Cross-Linking polymerization in two-dimensional assemblies: Effect of the reactive group site. Macromolecules 32:5519–5524
46. Regen SL et al (1984) Ghost vesicles. J Am Chem Soc 106:5756–5757
47. Lee JH, Danino D, Raghavan SB (2009) Polymerizable vesicles based on a single-tailed fatty acid surfactant: a simple route to robust nanocontainers. Langmuir 25:1566–1571
48. Kaler EW et al (2003) Structural fixation of spontaneous vesicles in aqueous mixtures of polymerizable anionic and cationic surfactants. Langmuir 19:10732–10738
49. Bordes R et al (2007) Novel polymerizable surfactants from 1:1 mixtures of alkylcarboxylic acids and norbornene methylenamine. Langmuir 23:7526–7530
50. DePierro MA (2006) Photopolymerization behavior and nanostructure development in lyotropic liquid crystals. Dissertation, The University of Iowa
51. Sisson TM et al (1996) Cross-linking polymerizations in two-dimensional assemblies. Macromolecules 29:8321–8329
52. McGrath KM, Drummond CJ (1996) Polymerization of liquid crystalline phases in binary surfactant/water systems. Coll Polym Sci 274:612–621
53. McGrath KM (1996) Polymerization of liquid crystalline phases in binary surfactant/water systems. Coll Polym Sci 274:399–409
54. Gin DL et al (2001) Polymerized lyotropic liquid crystals assemblies for materials applications. Acc Chem Res 34:973–980
55. Hatakeyama ES et al (2010) Nanoporous, bicontinuous cubic lyotropic liquid crystal networks via polymerizable gemini ammonium surfactants. Chem Mater 22:4525–5427
56. Mahantappa MK (2013) Polymerizable gemini dicarboxylate surfactants and lyotropic liquid crystals and membranes made therefrom. US patent 2013/0190417 A1, Jul. 25, 2013
57. Gabriel C et al (2012) Novel polymerizable surfactants platforms and uses thereof. US patent 20120211424 A1, 23 Jan 2012
58. Kwon YS et al (2010) Preparation of polymeric SWNT-liquid crystal composites using a polymerizable surfactant. Macromolecules. doi:10.1021/ma1003198
59. Gin DL et al (2006) Recent advances in the design of polymerizable lyotropic liquid-crystal assemblies for heterogeneous catalysis and selective separations. Adv Func Mat 16:865–878
60. Gin DL et al (2008) Polymerized lyotropic liquid crystal assemblies for membrane applications. Macromol Rapid Commun 29:367–389
61. Bara JE et al (2010) Thermotropic liquid crystal behavior of gemini imidazolium-based ionic amphiphiles. Liq Cryst 37:1587–1599
62. Bai Y, Guo J, Wei J (2012) The recent development of polymerizable lyotropic liquid crystal assemblies. Inf Rec Mater 1:6
63. Craspy D, Landfester K (2010) Miniemulsion polymerization as a versatile tool for the synthesis of functionalized polymers. Beilstein J Org Chem 6:1132–1148
64. Stoffer JO, Bone T (1983) Polymerization in water-in-oil microemulsion systems II: semi investigation of structure. Dispers Sci Technol 1:393–412
65. Attik SS, Thomas KJ (1981) Polymerized microemulsions. J Am Chem Soc 103:4279–4280
66. Gan LM et al (1995) Microporous polymeric materials from polymerization of zwitterionic microemulsions. Langmuir 11:3316–3320

Chapter 3
Polymerization Behavior of Surface-Active Monomers

As it was mentioned previously, the utilization of reactive surfmers permits to obtain polymeric colloids directly during polymerization and copolymerization reactions. The resulted colloids bear a range of important properties, namely the enhanced stability and functionalized interface of polymeric particles. The application of surfmers during the emulsion polymerization provides the facilities of controlling the size of latex particles and monitoring their aggregation stability [1]. This task could be also solved by immobilization of surface-active oligomers containing the fragments of reactive functional surfmers at interface of off-the-shelf polymeric colloidal systems. This approach allows us to create polymers with improved properties, latexes with "core–shell" particles morphology, to form grafted polymeric nanolayers on micro- and macrosurfaces. Moreover, when surface-active monomers are used, the polymerization reaction in micelles leads to high values of monomer conversion (usually higher than 90 %). Another practical importance of surfmers is connected with the synthesis of polyelectrolytes (via homo- and copolymerization) which have found applications in various fields of science and engineering [2]. One of the most rapidly and intensively developing tasks is the creation on their bases the carriers for the immobilization and delivering of biological and medical substances.

3.1 Emulsion Polymerization

Emulsion polymerization refers to a unique process employed for some radical chain polymerizations. It involves the polymerization of monomers in the form of emulsions. As it was already mentioned previously, the presence of surfactant during this process could cause a range of disadvantages for further application of emulsion polymers. Therefore, the employment of surfmers allows a certain number of benefits, namely the stability of resulted latexes, maintenance of adhesive properties, and introduction of functional group on the latex surface.

© The Author(s) 2014
M. Borzenkov and O. Hevus, *Surface Active Monomers*,
SpringerBriefs in Materials, DOI: 10.1007/978-3-319-08446-6_3

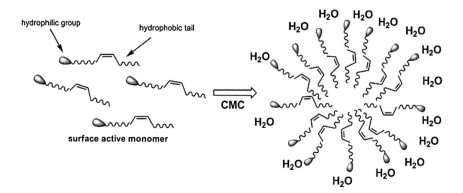

Scheme 3.1 Formation of micelles by surfmers in aqueous solutions

According to the general colloidal–chemical conceptions of the behavior surfactants in water, it could be assumed that in case of surfmers, the formation of molecule–micelle-associated species is observed at surfmer concentration in water above the CCM [2]. Many characteristics of the surfmer polymerization process in water are concerned with the formation of micelles [3]. The formation of micelles by surfmers in aqueous solutions is schematically shown in Scheme 3.1.

The scheme of the formation of polymeric dispersions during emulsion polymerization in the presence of surfmers has been already provided in Chap. 1. It was mentioned in previous chapters that reactivity, location of polymerizable fragment, and surface-active properties, which are governed by CMC, of surfmers are essential parameters for preparation latexes. Surfmers with high solubility in water could lead to its oligomerization in the aqueous phase and therefore to reduce the incorporation into latex structure. This process leads to lower stability of latex particles. High reactivity of polymerizable fragment could promote the homopolymerization of surfmer and, therefore, poor incorporation into latex particle, decreasing the particle stability.

In 1958, Freedman et al. reported about the synthesis of vinyl monomers, which also served as emulsifying agents [4]. The first report of polymerization of surface-active monomer was made in the publication of Bistline et al. [5]. Since these times, surfmers have been paid much attention. Great variety of surfmers with different polymerizable fragments located in various parts of molecule was synthesized for the purpose of stabilizing micelles and vesicles during the polymerization. The polymerization processes in the presence of surfmers are studied by research groups worldwide. A vast amount of publications exists in the field of polymerization of surfmers. A number of publications [6–10] and well-grounded reviews [11–14] in this field should be mentioned.

One of the first researches devoted to the polymerization of nonionic surfmers was reported by research group of Ottewill [15]. The authors synthesized and applied for obtaining polystyrene latexes macromonomer containing polyethylene oxide chain. The resulted latexes were resistant to fluctuation caused by adding electrolyte. The utilization of macromonomers containing polyethylene oxide chain was evaluated as one of the most suitable techniques for obtaining branched polymers with well-defined structure [16, 17]. The impact of lengths of alkylic and polyethylene oxide chains on the rate of polymerization was studied for monomers with the following structure: $R–O–(CH_2CH_2O)_n–CH_2–C_6H_4–CH=CH_2$ [18]. It was found that the highest polymerization rate was achieved in case of n = 15–20.

In the earliest surveys devoted to the preparation of latexes in the presence of anionic surfmers, sodium-9 (and 10) acrylamido stearate was applied [19]. The corresponding latexes with polymerizable surfactant immobilized onto particle surface were shown improved mechanical and electrical resistance [20, 21]. The copolymerization of sodium acrylaminoundecanoate with styrene and butyl acrylate aimed at obtaining latexes with carboxylic groups onto their surface was described in paper published in 1990 [22]. The impact of nature of anionic surfmer-polymerizable fragment was studied [23]. Among the earliest publications about emulsion polymerization in the presence of cationic surfmers, the works of Tauer et al. and Egorov [2, 24] should be mentioned. The emulsion polymerization of styrene, vinyl acetate, and chloroprene in the presence of cationic surfmers obtained by the reaction of alkylic esters of bromoacetic acid with tertiary unsaturated amines was reported [25]. The application of N-decylaceto-2-methyl-5vinylpyridine bromide for emulsion polymerization of styrene, butyl acrylate, and chloroprene initiated by 2,2'azoisobutyronitrile or potassium persulfate was reported [26]. The resulted latexes showed a high resistance to the influence of electrolytes, temperatures and redispersion. The emulsion polymerization of styrene and the properties of resulted latexes in the presence of a range of maleic and (meth)acrylic surfmers were reported in the following papers [27–30]. The results of radical polymerization and copolymerization of alkyl bromide salts of 2-dimethylaminoethyl methacrylate having a different alkyl chain length in various solvents giving micellar and isotropic solutions aimed at obtaining an insight into micellar polymerization were summarized in the publication of Nagai [31]. It was found that the monomer micellization of the cationic surface-active monomers at concentrations far above their critical micelle concentration leads to significant increases in the rate of polymerization and the molecular weight of the resulting polymers for both aqueous and inverse micellar solutions and the tendency toward alternation of the copolymerization for aqueous micellar systems, whereas it has little influence on the tacticity of the resulting polymers [31].

In the previous paragraphs, the main publications devoted to the polymerization in the presence of surface-active monomers until 2000 were briefly highlighted. The following part of this chapter compactly focuses on recent publications in this field.

Hybrid organic–inorganic phases composed of a surface-active monomer and sulfopropyl methacrylate, incorporated within the lamellar structure of layered double hydroxides and its subsequent polymerization, were reported in the paper published in 2004 [32]. The studies suggested that the oxygen molecules may act as an external initiator of polymerization. Further studies indicated that the polymerization of surfmer was kinetically limited. Cationic maleic dialkyl surfmer containing 12 atoms of carbon in hydrophobic part was synthesized and applied for emulsion copolymerization with other monomers [33]. A series of new polymerizable nonionic and ionic surfactants (surfmers) with amide groups on both sides of the C = C double bonds have been prepared upon reaction of maleic isoimide carrying a long alkyl chain (or a benzyl group) with a hydrophilic amine derivative. They have been engaged in batch emulsion polymerization of styrene and semi-batch seeded copolymerization of styrene and butyl acrylate, giving stable latexes during the polymerization process and upon extraction with ethanol, showing a high rate of incorporation at the particle surface [34]. Novel surface-active monomers and initiators were synthesized by successive treatment of cumylsuccinic anhydride with 3-*tert*-butylperoxy-3-methyl-1-butanol or poly(propylene glycol) acrylate and 1,3-propane sultone with triethylamine. The synthesized compounds were shown to be suitable reactive surfactants for obtaining styrene latexes [35]. A surface-active monomer, polyisobutylene-succinimide pentamine, was used as a stabilizer for synthesizing polyurea nanocapsules with aqueous core via polyaddition at inverse miniemulsion droplet interface [36]. Due to the presence of amine groups in the surfmer molecule, it is covalently incorporated into the polymeric interfacial layer after reaction, resulting in more compact (less permeable) capsule shell. The influence of the stabilizer and the monomer concentration on the shell thickness, colloidal stability, and average capsule size were studied. The properties and stability of latexes obtained in the presence of surface-active monomers are also well described in the publication of Volkov and Rodionova [37]. Also, the utilization of surfmers during emulsion polymerization and stability of resulted colloids were described in the publication of Chern [38]. The behavior of anionic and cationic maleic surfmers containing a benzyl or vinylbenzyl hydrophobic tail in the emulsion polymerization process of styrene was studied [39]. It was shown in this publication that that the utilization of synthesized surfmers for emulsion polymerization of styrene allows obtaining stable latex particles with narrow size distribution. The concentration of surfmer incorporated during polymerization allows controlling the particle size.

It has been already mentioned in previous chapters that a various types of surface-active monomers have been synthesized by the research group at Department of Organic Chemistry of Lviv Polytechnic National University. Therefore, it is necessary to provide a brief description of their polymerization properties.

The synthesized maleate surfmers containing hydrophilic, polyethylene glycolic, propanesulfonic, and triethylamine units, lipophilic, alkylic, fluoroalkylic, olygomethylsiloxanic, and di-tert-peroxide group and cationic acrylate surfmers were copolymerized with styrene, the parameters of copolymerization were studied, and the characteristics of resulted copolymers were described [1, 40–42]. It was found that that synthesized monomers are capable for free radical copolymerization with styrene. At the same time, the peroxide-containing surfmers during the copolymerization preserve the di-tert-peroxide group [42]. The copolymerization in solution and emulsion copolymerization of synthesized saccharide-containing surface-active monomers [43] with vinyl acetate, N-vinylpyrrolidone, peroxide-containing monomer 5-tert-butylperoxy-5-methyl-2-hexene-3-yne (VEP) [44], and styrene was performed. The main goal was aimed at obtaining biologically tolerant oligomeric carriers of pharmaceutical substances. The saccharide-containing monomers have been shown to be capable of copolymerization with the formation of copolymers bearing saccharide moieties in side polymer chains. The synthesized peroxide-containing saccharide surface active have been shown to be capable of initiation of polymerization of aqueous emulsion of styrene with formation of stable aqueous polystyrene dispersions.

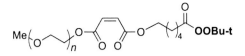

Scheme 3.2 The chemical structure of nonionic surfmer applied as comonomer initiator of styrene emulsion polymerization

Scheme 3.3 The chemical structure of surface-active monomer with phosphate group

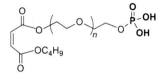

The polymerization of styrene in the presence of peroxide-containing nonionic maleate surfmer with the structure displayed in Scheme 3.2 was studied [45]. The singularity of process was that during the copolymerization, the peroxide-containing surfmer acted as comonomer and also as initiator at the same time.

The styrene conversion of 80–85 % was achieved in 6–7 h. The increasing of surfmer content leads to increasing of polymerization rate content as it is known that increasing of emulsifier content leads to increasing of polymerization rate [46]. The copolymerization of phosphate containing surfmer with N-vinylpyrrolidone and with N-vinylpyrrolidone and VEP was also performed [47]. The chemical structure of corresponding phosphate monomer is shown in Scheme 3.3.

The resulted copolymer surfmer-VEP- N-vinylpyrrolidone was applied as surface-active macroinitiator of styrene emulsion polymerization led to the formation of stable polymeric colloidal systems.

3.2 Polymerization in Microemulsion

According to IUPAC definition, microemulsion is a stable system with dispersed domain diameter varying approximately from 1 to 100 nm, but usually 10–50 nm. Polymerization reactions that are performed in a globular phase of microemulsions yield well-defined, narrowly distributed microlatex particles [48]. Their size is typically one order of magnitude smaller compared with that obtained by standard emulsion polymerization. Polymers can be synthesized in a miniemulsion system in the dispersed phase, at the interface of the droplets, or in the continuous phase. The concept of polymerization in microemulsion has developed recently since 1980 due to the attractive features of microemulsions [38, 49]. Diameters of polymer particles formed during microemulsion polymerization are usually in range 10–50 nm [50]. Microemulsion polymerization was applied for the synthesis of highly functionalized nanoparticles [51]. The main drawback of microemulsion polymerization is the low monomer content. The employment of surfmers therefore was investigated with the aim to increase the final polymer content. Moreover, the units of surfmer are incorporated in the structure of final polymer. Surface-active monomers are successfully incorporated into the microemulsion polymerization as the utilization of these compounds can solve a range of problems connected with the application of non-polymerizable surfactants and to obtain highly functionalized nanoparticles [11, 51, 52]. Larpent et al. [53] prepared styrene-in-water microemulsions using sodium dodecyl sulfate and polymerizable cosurfactants such as hydroxyalkyl acrylates or methacrylates. Polymerization led to well-defined highly functionalized nanoparticles in the 15–25 nm diameter range. Tieke et al. [28], however, reported about direct employment of surfmers as polymerizable cosurfactants. Styrene and 11-((acryloyloxy)undecyl) trimethylammonium bromide formed transparent microemulsions without addition of any cosurfactant. The polymerization resulted in nanolatex particles approximately 21 nm in diameter. Pileni et al. [54] proposed a strategy for the synthesis of latex nanoparticles in the size range 2–5 nm. The paper by Capek and Chern [55] presents a review in the field of radical polymerization of conventional monomers and surface-active monomers in direct miniemulsion systems focusing particle nucleation mechanisms and the common and different features between the classical emulsion and finer miniemulsion polymerization systems. An interesting review of an overview of the different polymer syntheses within the miniemulsion droplets is presented in the publication of Crespy and Landfester [56]. The application of various surfmers in radical microemulsion polymerization is described in this review. Li et al. [57] reported about the preparation of ultrafiltration membranes by direct polymerization of bicontinuous microemulsions. For the preparation of these microemulsions, the surface-active monomers, namely ((acryloyloxy)undecyl)trimethylammonium bromide and ((acryloyloxy)undecyl)dimethylammonio acetate, were used. The uniqueness of the resulted microemulsion systems was that all organic components can readily be copolymerized at room temperature using a redox initiator.

The cationic reactive surfmers were covalently anchored on the surfaces of the formed particles, as indicated by a positive zeta potential. Core–shell silicone acrylic miniemulsions with 3-methacryloxypropyl trimethoxysilane in the shell were prepared with the assistance of polymerizable maleate surfactant [58]. The impact of monomer concentration on particle size and viscosity was studied.

Miniemulsion systems were found to be suitable to conduct controlled radical polymerizations [59] including atom transfer radical polymerization (ATRP) and reversible addition–fragmentation transfer (RAFT). Therefore, these aspects are reviewed in the following sections.

3.3 Radical Polymerization and Atom Transfer Radical Polymerization

Radical polymerization is considered as one of the most common reactions to synthesize polymers. This is a chain polymerization in which the kinetic chain carriers are radicals. It is known that the mechanism of the corresponding polymerization can be described in four stages: initiation, propagation, transfer, and termination. One of the first examples of radical polymerization of surfmers was the polymerization of the sodium salts of the allyl esters of α-sulfopalmitic and α-sulfostearic acids [5]. Their radical polymerization yielded water-soluble polymers with an average degree of polymerization of 10. A study of the radical polymerization of methacryloyloxy-alkylammonium salts with an alkyl fragment of equal length showed that in certain cases, the effects associated with the ionic character of the surfmers may have a greater influence on the polymerization kinetics in the solution than the association phenomenon [60]. Processes of structurization were studied in radical polymerization of N,N-dimethyl-N-methacroylethyl-alkylacetylammonium bromides or chlorides in toluene, initiated by thermal decomposition of azoisobutyronitrile [61]. The formation of primary reversed micelles was observed, together with the formation of anisotropic secondary micelles in the course of their accumulation. It was found that polymerization only occurs in the primary micelles and that the polymerization rate decreases for monomers containing a bulky counterion, or by introducing water into the system. Radical copolymerizations of anionic surface-active monomer and sodium di(10-undecenyl)sulfosuccinate with electron-accepting monomers and vinyl monomers were studied in water, n-hexane, and dioxane, giving aqueous micellar solution, reverse micellar solution, and isotropic solution, respectively [62]. The copolymerizations of this surfmer with hydrophobic diethyl fumarate in aqueous micellar solution afforded the copolymer in relatively high yields as compared to those for the copolymerizations in reverse micellar and isotropic solutions. On the other hand, the copolymerization with hydrophilic fumaronitrile in isotropic solution proceeded at a higher rate than that in aqueous and reverse micellar solutions. In the later publication, Nagai [31] reported about the results on radical polymerization and copolymerization of alkyl bromide salts of 2-dimethylaminoethyl methacrylate having a different alkyl chain length in various solvents giving micellar and isotropic solutions. The monomer micellization of the cationic surface-active monomers at concentrations far above their CMC led to significant increases in the rate of polymerization and the molecular weight of the resulting polymers for both aqueous and inverse micellar solutions. The previously mentioned publication of Capek and Chern [55] presents a review of the current literature in the field of radical polymerization of conventional monomers and surface-active monomers in direct miniemulsion systems. Besides a short introduction about some kinetic aspects of radical polymerization in direct emulsion, miniemulsion, and microemulsion systems, the authors mainly focused on the particle nucleation mechanisms and the common and different features between the classical emulsion and finer miniemulsion polymerization systems. Pich et al. [63] reported about monofluorooctyl surface-active maleate monomer that was synthesized and applied for radical polymerization in miniemulsions.

Polymer modification of colloidal silica by radical copolymerization of surfmers containing terminated vinyl group was investigated [56]. Radical copolymerization of amide ammonium monomer and ammonium-type cross-linker (monomer) using an initiator of 2,2′-azobis(2-amidinopropane) dihydrochloride on colloidal silica successfully led to the formation of monodispersed cross-linked polymer/SiO$_2$ composites, which were stable in organic solvents. Cho et al. [64] in a paper published in 2010 described the synthesis and preparation of novel acrylic

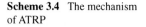

Scheme 3.4 The mechanism
of ATRP

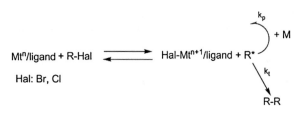

surface-active monomers. The resulted monomers were polymerized by the radical polymerization, using benzoyl peroxide as a catalyst. The molecular weights of the polymers prepared under different experimental conditions were in the range from 20,000 to 30,000 g/mol.

In the first part of current subchapter, the some aspects of radical polymerization of surfmers were briefly reviewed. The second part is devoted to the application of surfmers in atom transfer radical polymerization.

Atom transfer radical polymerization (ATRP) is among the most effective and most widely used methods of controlled radical polymerization. ATRP was developed in 1995 independently by Wang and Matyjaszewski and Kato et al. [65–67] as an expansion of transition metal catalyzed atom transfer radical addition (ATRA). In this technique, atom transfer from an organic halide to a transition metal complex occurs to "activate" organic radicals which are then quickly "deactivated" by back transfer of the atom from the transition metal to the organic radical species [68]. The stages of ATRP reaction are as follows: initiation, equilibrium with dormant species, and propagation. The number of growing polymer chains is determined by the initiator. Organic halides that are similar in the organic framework as the propagating radical are often chosen as initiators. The mechanism of ATRP is schematically shown in Scheme 3.4.

The advantages of ATRP are numerous: Catalytic amounts of transition metal complexes are used; employment of commercially available complexes; a large range of polymers can be polymerized (with the exception of unprotected acids); end functionalization is very simple; a large range of temperatures can be employed [68]. The limitations of ATRP include that the transition metal complex must often be removed from the product, and the acidic monomers require protection [68].

The ATRP of neutral 2-hydroxyethyl methacrylate and cationic 2-(N,N,N-trimethylammonio)ethyl methacrylate triflate and 2-(N,N,N-dimethylethylammonio) ethyl methacrylate bromide were described in the works by Min, Armes and Dubois [69–71]. Bortolamei et al. [72] in their work published in 2011 focused on the polymerization of oligo(ethylene glycol) methyl ether methacrylate in water with a $Cu^{II/I}$/TPMA (TPMA = tris(2-pyridylmethyl)amine) catalyst system and illustrated that many of the drawbacks typically associated with conventional aqueous ATRP could be overcome. This specific polymerization of this monomer in water with a $Cu^{II/I}$/TPMA catalyst was selected for study as the final polymer would be biocompatible and conducted such a reaction in water as the primary solvent was a critical step in defining conditions for conducting ATRP under biologically compatible conditions. A well-controlled polymerization of oligo(ethylene oxide) methyl ether methacrylate was conducted with 100–300 ppm of a copper catalyst with tris(2-pyridylmethyl)amine ligand in the presence of an excess of ligand and an excess of halide salts at room temperature [73].

A surface-active monomer 11'-(methacryloyloxy)-undecyl(trimethyl)ammonium bromide was synthesized and used as a stabilizer and comonomer for activator generated by electron transfer atom transfer radical polymerization (AGET ATRP) of n-butyl methacrylate in emulsion [74]. This reactive "surfactant" was applied in a continuous two-step microemulsion to emulsion technique. Stable polymer latexes with size ranging from 40 to 200 nm were obtained by adjusting the amount of reactive surfactant introduced to the system. The surfactant concentration could be decreased to as low as 1.3 wt % in the final emulsion (5.9 wt % vs monomer), while still maintaining good colloidal stability. The cationic reactive surfactants were covalently anchored on the surfaces of the formed particles, as indicated by a positive zeta potential. In addition, a well-controlled polymerization process was achieved by ATRP, as evidenced by the smooth increase in molecular weight of the polymer chains as the polymerization progressed and by the formation of polymers with preserved chain-end functionalities.

In the recent years, polymeric ionic liquids or poly(ionic liquid)s (PILs) were found to take an enabling role in polymeric chemistry and material science [75]. PILs combine the unique properties of ionic liquids with the flexibility and the properties of macromolecular architectures and provide novel properties and functions that are of huge potential in a multitude of applications. Living/controlled radical polymerization of IL monomer, 2-(1-butylimidazolium-3-yl)ethyl methacrylate tetrafluoroborate, by ATRP was firstly reported by Shen et al. [76]. With copper(I) chloride/2,2'-bipyridine as the catalyst system and trichloroacetate, CCl_4, or ethyl-chlorophenylacetate as initiator, this monomer was polymerized at 60 °C with first-order kinetics with respect to monomer concentration. Later, this research group extended this technique to styrenic IL monomers of 1-(4-vinylbenzyl)-3-butyl imidazolium tetrafluoroborate and 1-(4-vinylbenzyl)-3-butyl imidazolium hexafluorophosphate [76]. The polymerization was well controlled and exhibited living characteristics when Cu(I)Br/2,2'-bipyridine was used as catalyst system.

3.4 Reversible Addition-Fragmentation Chain Transfer Polymerization

RAFT polymerization is a reversible deactivation radical polymerization (RDRP) and one of the more versatile methods for providing living characteristics to radical polymerization. RAFT polymerization is a form of living radical polymerization involving conventional free radical polymerization of a substituted monomer in the presence of a suitable chain transfer (RAFT) reagent. Advantages of RAFT polymerization include the following [77].

- The ability to control polymerization of most monomers polymerizable by radical polymerization. These include (meth)acrylates, (meth)acrylamides, acrylonitrile, styrenes, dienes, and vinyl monomers.

- Tolerance of unprotected functionality in monomer and solvent (e.g., OH, NR_2, COOH, $CONR_2$, SO_3H). Polymerizations can be carried out in aqueous or protic media.
- Compatibility with reaction conditions (e.g., bulk, organic, or aqueous solution, emulsion, miniemulsion, suspension).
- Ease of implementation and inexpensive relative to competitive technologies.

The mechanism of RAFT polymerization is described in detail in a range of publications [77–79]. Actually, in article published [79] in 1998, a novel "living" free radical polymerization technique, RAFT process, was firstly reported. Briefly, the mechanism of RAFT polymerization includes the following initiation: As in conventional free radical polymerization, the radical reversibly adds onto the chain transfer agent to form an intermediate radical, which can fragment to liberate a reinitiating group and form a new dormant chain. The new radical reinitiates polymerization by reaction on monomers. The rapid establishment of this reversible addition–fragmentation equilibrium allows for control over molecular weight and molecular weight distribution, although irreversible termination reactions still occur, mainly due to the free radical introduced initially to initiate polymerization [78]. The RAFT process involves free radical polymerization in the presence of dithioesters, xanthates, and trithiocarbonates as transfer agents.

The polymerization of surfmers by RAFT polymerization process is briefly described in this subchapter. The application of RAFT in miniemulsion polymerization stabilized by surfmers promotes to obtain polymeric latexes with controlled molecular weight and with properties obtained from the employment of surfmers. Matahwa et al. [80] in their paper published in 2005 reported about cationic and anionic surfmers, which are 11-methacryloyloxyundecan-1-yl trimethyl ammonium bromide and sodium 11-methacryloyloxyundecan-1-yl sulfate, respectively. These surfmers were synthesized and used to stabilize particles in miniemulsion polymerization. A comparative study of classical cationic and anionic surfactants and the two surfmers was conducted with respect to the reaction rates and molecular weight distributions of the formed polymers. The reversible addition–fragmentation chain transfer process was used in the miniemulsion polymerization reactions to control the molecular weight distribution. 4-Cyano-4-(thiobenzoyl) sulfonyl pentanoic acid was synthesized as RAFT agent. The reaction rates of the surfmer-stabilized miniemulsion polymerization of styrene and methyl methacrylate were similar (in most cases) to those of the classical-surfactant-stabilized miniemulsion polymerizations. The final particle sizes were also similar for polystyrene latexes stabilized by the surfmers and classical surfactants. However, poly(methyl methacrylate) latexes stabilized by the surfmers had larger particle sizes than latexes stabilized by classical surfactants. The advances in the use of the RAFT process including the application of surfmers in RAFT polymerization process are described in the publication of McLeary and Klumperman [81]. In the recent publication, FitzGerald et al. [82] and coworkers used RAFT to polymerize the T-type surface-active monomer α,ω-methacryloylund ecyltrimethylammonium bromide to various degrees of polymerization and investigated how its self-assembly was affected. Small-angle neutron scattering showed that the interchain aggregation into micelles with an approximately constant number of surfmer equivalents occured at low degrees of polymerization, but that micelle elongation occured when the degree of polymerization exceeds a critical value. In this regime, interchain aggregation gives way to intrachain assembly into unimolecular or "unimer" micelles. As with conventional cationic surfactant solutions, addition of salicylate produced long, wormlike micelles containing many amphiphilic polymer chains at all degrees of polymerization. Oscillatory rheology revealed a transition from scission- to reptation-dominated relaxation as increasing polymer chain length also increases the distance between potential scission points. The measured relaxation times lay in the range of hundreds to a few seconds—thus demonstrating the rapidly equilibrating nature of these micellar systems even at the highest degrees of polymerization achieved. Cationic polymerizable surfactants based on styrene with fluorocarbon chains and their hydrocarbon analogues were synthesized and copolymerized to give micellar polymers of the polysoap type [83]. Characteristically, the fluorocarbon polymers showed a higher tendency for self-organization, but also much less mobile hydrophobic associations in aqueous media than their hydrocarbon counterparts. In contrast to statistical terpolymers of similar average composition, block copolymers made of a fluorocarbon polysoap block and a hydrocarbon polysoap block via the radical addition–fragmentation chain transfer method gave rise to not only microphase separation between the hydrophilic polar parts and the hydrophobic apolar parts of the macromolecules, but also seemed to be able to undergo additional microphase separation between hydrophobic domains made of fluorocarbon chains and those made of hydrocarbon chains, at least in the solid state.

Novel family of methacrylate surfmers was synthesized, and their RAFT polymerization in the presence of 2-phenylprop-2-yl dithiobenzoate as RAFT agent was studied [84].

In the previous subchapter, it has been already mentioned about significant properties of poly(ionic liquid)s (PILs) and application of ATRP technique to synthesize PILs. Compared with ATRP, RAFT polymerization of IL monomers comes with a short delay [75]. Gnanou et al. [85] demonstrated the synthesis of PIL-based double hydrophilic block copolymers by sequential RAFT polymerization of methacryloyl-based IL monomer and acryl amide or methacrylic acid. Shen et al. [86] described the preparation of diblock copolymers by sequential RAFT polymerization of N-2-thiazolylmethacrylamide and 2-(1-butylimidazolium-3-yl) ethyl methacrylate tetrafluoroborate. During the RAFT polymerization of methacryloyl-based IL monomers introduced by corresponding by these authors the imidazolium cation is well-separated from the polymerizing unit by an alkyl spacer in the monomers. The radical polymerization proceeded without or with fewer disturbances by the imidazolium ring. Yuan et al. [87] performed the RAFT polymerization of four 1-vinylimidazolium IL monomers possessing different alkyl substitutes and anions. It was found that in the chain extension reaction, the reactivity of an IL monomer bearing dicyanamide anion was significantly lower than that of monomers with halides due to large anion size.

Novel approach for the synthesis of core–shell polystyrene nanoparticles by living hydrophilic polymer consisting of thiocarbonyl thio end group was reported in a paper published in Journal of Colloid and Interface Science in 2011 [88]. The surfactant-free emulsion polymerization of styrene in the presence of macro-RAFT agent was carried out to synthesize stable latex particles with smaller particle size. A macro-RAFT agent was prepared by homopolymerization of sodium styrene sulfonate in aqueous phase by using dithioester as chain transfer agent.

3.5 Synthesis of Polyelectrolyte Polymers

The synthesis of polyelectrolyte polymers is another important focus of many researches due to their properties and successful application in biology [89–91]. Polyelectrolyte polymers are water-soluble polymers carrying ionic charge along the polymer chain, and depending upon the charge, these polymers are anionic or cationic. Therefore, the utilization of cationic and anionic surfmers is considered as a prospective strategy for obtaining novel polyelectrolyte polymers.

New cationic and anionic polyelectrolytes were synthesized by bulk radical copolymerization of 2-hydroxyethyl methacrylate with 2-methacryloyloxyethyltrimethyl ammonium chloride or 2-acrylamido-2-methylpropane-sulfonic acid monomers [92]. Swelling studies on synthesized copolymers showed a high water content in the swollen state and a "smart behavior" upon changes in external stimuli (pH and ionic strength). Free radical homopolymerization of tail-type cationic surface-active monomers proceeded very rapidly in water as a result of organization in the micelle to afford the corresponding amphiphilic cationic polyelectrolyte with $M_w = 3.63 \times 10^6$ and 23 nm hydrodynamic radius [93]. The vesicular polymerization of two-tail surfmers, dicetyldimethylammonium 4-vinyl benzoate and dicetyldimethylammonium 3,5-vinyl benzoate, which led to the formation polyelectrolyte chains, was reported [94]. The flocculation in mixtures of cationic polyelectrolytes and anionic surfactant was reported in the paper by Vincent B [95].

The polymerization behavior of surfmers obtained on the basis of derivatives of hydroxy carboxylic acid [96] was also studied. Hence, the solution copolymerization of synthesized surfmers with peroxide-containing monomer VEP and N-vinylpyrrolidone was carried out. The general structure of synthesized surface-active copolymers is shown in Scheme 3.5.

The resulted copolymers are water soluble and reduce surface tension at aqueous solution–air interface. The incorporation of units of surface-active monomers into copolymer structure increases their surface activity in comparison with binary copolymer VEP–N-vinylpyrrolidone. It was also found that incorporation of units of ionic surfmers into structure of VEP–N-vinylpyrrolidone macromolecules provides the polyelectrolyte properties, namely the capability to form interpolyelectrolyte complex (IPEC) with oppositely charged polymers. Therefore, the study of IPEC formation between model copolymers and synthesized copolymers with surfmer fragments is an effective technique for the estimation of their ability to bind biopolymers, particularly nucleic acids. Obtained results indicated the formation of stable IPEC during the interaction between model and synthesized oppositely charged polyelectrolytes.

Scheme 3.5 General structure of surface-active copolymers containing links of novel surface-active monomers

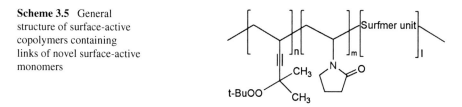

In this chapter, the application and advantages of employment of surfmers at various polymerization processes including recently developed miniemulsion and ATRP and RAFT techniques were briefly overviewed. The introduction of surfmers in these processes has a range of significant advantages in comparison with traditional surfactants.

References

1. Hevus OI (2010) Funkcionalni poverhnevo-aktuvni peroxidy I monomery yak reagentu dlia oderjannia reakciynozdatnuh modufikatoriv poverhni (Functional surface active peroxides and monomers for creation of reactive surface modifiers). Dissertation, Lviv Polytechnic National University
2. Egorov VV, Zubov VP (1987) Radical polymerization in the associated species of iono-genic surface active monomers in water. Russ Chem Rev (Translated from Uspekhi Khimii) 56:2076–2097
3. Martin W, Ringsdorf J, Thuning D (1977) Polymerization of organized systems. Midl Macr Monogr 3:175
4. Freedman HH, Mason JP, Medalia AI (1958) Polysoaps—II: the preparation of vinyl soaps. J Am Chem Soc 23:76–82
5. Bistline RG et al (1956) Synthetic detergents from animal fats. VI. Polymerizable esters of α-sulfonated fatty acids. J Am Oil Chem Soc 33:44–45
6. Nagai K et al (1985) Polymerization of surface-active monomers. I. Micellization and polymerization of higher alkyl salts of dimethylaminoethyl methacrylate. J Polym Sci Part A: Polym Chem Ed 23:1221–1230
7. Hamid SM, Sherrington DC (1987) Novel quaternary ammonium amphiphilic (meth) acrylates: 1. Synthesis, melting and interfacial behaviour. Polymer 28:325–331
8. Fontanille M, Guyot A (1987) Recent advances in mechanistic and synthetic aspect of polymerization. Reidel, Dordrecht
9. Maniruzzaman M, Kawaguchi S, Ito K (2000) Micellar copolymerization of styrene with poly(ethylene oxide) macromonomer in water: approach to unimolecular nanoparticles via pseudo-living radical polymerization. Macromolecules 33:1583–1592
10. Regen SL, Czech B, Singh A (1980) Polymerized vesicles. J Am Chem Soc 102:6638–6640
11. Summers M, Eastoe J (2003) Application of polymerizable surfactants. Adv Coll Int Sci 100–102:137–152
12. Jönsson B (1998) Surfactants and polymers in aqueous solution. Wiley, Chichester
13. Aida T, Tajima K (2000) Controlled polymerization with constrained geometries. Chem Commun 24:2399–2412
14. Guyot A (2003) Polymerizable surfactants. In: Holmberg K (ed) Novel surfactants. Preparation, application and biodegradability. Marcel Dekker, New York
15. Ottewill RH, Satgurunathan R (1987) Non-ionic lattices in aqueous media. part 1. synthesis and characterization. J Colloid Polym Sci 265:845–852

16. Ito K (1988) Polymeric design by macromonomer technique. Prog Polym Sci 23:581–620
17. Ito K, Kawaguchi S (1999) Poly(macromonomers): Homo- and Copolymerization. Adv Polym Sci 142:129–178
18. Ito K et al (1991) Poly(ethylene oxide) macromonomers. 7. Micellar polymerization in water. Macromolecules 24:2348–2354
19. Greene BW, Sheetz DP, Filer TD (1970) In situ polymerization of surface-active agents on latex particles II. The mechanical stability of styrene/butadiene latexes. J Colloid Interface Sci 32:90–95
20. Greene BW, Sheetz DP (1970) In situ polymerization of surface-active agents on latex Particles II. The mechanical stability of styrene/butadiene latexes. J Colloid Interface Sci 32:96–100
21. Greene BW, Saunders FL (1970) In situ polymerization of surface-active agents on latex Particles III. The electrolyte stability of styrene/butadiene latexes. J Colloid Interface Sci 33:393–404
22. Guillaume JL, Pichot C, Guillot J (1990) Emulsifier-free emulsion copolymerization of styrene and butyl acrylate. III. Kinetic studies in the presence of a surface active comonomer, the sodium acrylamido undecanoate. J Polym Sci Part A: Polym Chem Ed 28:137–152
23. Schoonbrood HAS et al (1997) Reactive surfactants in heterophase polymerization. 7. Emulsion copolymerization mechanism involving three anionic polymerizable surfactants (surfmers) with styrene-butyl acrylate-acrylic acid. Macromolecules 30:6024–6033
24. Tauer K et al (1988) Neuere Entwicklungen bei der Synthese von Polymerdispersionen. Plaste Kautsch 35(373):378
25. Orlov YN (1985) Radicalnaia polymerizacia poverhnostno-aktivnyh monomerov v vodnyh emulsijah I dispersiah (Radical polymerization of surface active monomers in aqueous emulsions and dispersions). Dissertation, Moscow State University
26. Maliukova EB et al (1991) Emulsionnaya sopolimerizacia vinilovuh I dienovuh monomerov s poverhnostno-aktivnymi somonomerami (Emulsion copolymerization of vinyl and dienic monomers with surface active comonomers). High mol compd 33:1469–1475
27. Cochin D, Laschewsky A, Nallet F (1997) Emulsion polymerization of styrene using conventional, polymerizable, and polymeric surfactants. Comp Study Macromolecules 30:2278–2287
28. Dreja M, Tieke B (1996) Microemulsions with polymerizable surfactants. γ-ray induced copolymerization of styrene and 11-(acryloyloxy)-undecyl-(trimethyl)-ammonium bromide in three-component cationic microemulsion. Macromol Rapid Com 17:825–833
29. Abele S et al (1997) Reactive surfactants in heterophase polymerization. 10. Characterization of the surface activity of new polymerizable surfactants derived from maleic anhydride. Langmuir 13:176–181
30. Abele S et al (1999) Cationic and zwitterionic polymerizable surfactants: quaternary ammonium dialkyl maleates. 1. Synthesis and characterization. Langmuir 15:1033–1044
31. Nagai K (1994) Polymerization of surface active monomers and applications. Macromolecular Symposia 84:29–36
32. Swanson CR, Besse JP, Leroux F (2004) Polymerization of sulfopropyl methacrylate, a surface active monomer, within layered double hydroxide. Chem Mater 16:5512–5517
33. Yang SF et al (2005) St-Ba copolymer emulsions prepared by using novel cationic maleic dialkyl polymerizable emulsifier. Eur Polymer J 41:2973–2979
34. Klimenkovsa I, Zhukovskaa I, Uzulinaa I, Zicmanis A (2003) Maleic diamide polymerizable surfactants. Applications in emulsion polymerization. C R Chim 6:1295–1304
35. Hevus I, Pikh Z (2007) Novel surfactants for creating reactive polymers. Macromolec Symposia 1:103–108
36. Rosenbauer EM, Landfester K, Musyanovych A (2009) Surface active monomer as a stabilizer for polyurea nanocapsules synthesized via interfacial polyaddition in inverse miniemulsion. Langmuir 25:12084–12091
37. Volkov VA, Rodionova RV (2006) Synthesis and properties synthetic polymer latexes with copolymerized emulsifiers. Fibre Chem 38:259–364
38. Chern CS (2006) Emulsion polymerization mechanisms and kinetics. Prog Polym Sci 31:443–486

39. Mekki S et al (2010) Synthesis of new anionic and cationic polymerizable surfactants for emulsion polymerization of styrene. Marcomol Symp 296:100–106
40. Kohut AM, Hevus OI, Voronov SA (2004) Synthesis and properties of 4-(ω-methoxyoligodi methylsiloxanyl)butylmaleate; a new surfmer. J Appl Polymer Sci 93:310–313
41. Kohut AM (2006) Sintez i vlastuvosti poverhnevo-aktuvnuh monomeriv i peroxydiv (Synthesis and properties of surface active monomers and peroxides). Dissertation, Lviv Polytechnic National University
42. Kohut A et al (2007) Macroinitiators on the basis of new peroxide surface active monomers. Chem Chem Technol 1:83–86
43. Vuytsyk L et al (2008) Biosumisni gidrozoli nanochastunok zolota z obolonkou na osnovi sacharudovmisnogo oligomernogo surfactanty (Biocompatible gold nanoparticles covered with saccharide containing oligomeric surfactant). Nanostructurnoe materialovedenie (Mater Sci Nanostruct) 12:1109–1118
44. Zaichenko O et al (2008) Novel functional nanoscale composites on the basis of oligoperoxide surfactants: syntheses and biomedical applications. Biotechnology 1:82–94
45. Borzenkov MM, Hevus OI (2012) Novel peroxide containing maleate surface active monomers for obtaining reactive polymers. Macromolecular Symposia 315:60–65
46. Borzenkov M, Hevus O (2013) Synthesis and properties of novel surface active monomers containing phosphate group. In: Abstracts of European Polymer Congress EPF-2013, Pisa, Italy, 16–21. June, 2013
47. Arshady R (1992) Suspension, emulsion and dispersion polymerization: a methodological survey. Colloid Polym Sci 270:717–732
48. Antonietti M (1994) Polymerization in microemulsions of natural surfactants and protein functionalization of the particles. Langmuir 10:2498–24500
49. Moon JM (2009) Modification of monodisperse colloidal silica by radical copolymerization of cationic surface active vinyl monomers. Polym J 41:208–213
50. Gupta B, Gingh H (1992) Polymerization in microemulsion systems. Polym Plast Technol Eng 31:635–658
51. Pavel FM (2004) Microemulsion polymerization. J Dis Sci Technol 25:1–16
52. Slomkowski S et al (2011) Terminology of polymers and polymerization processes in dispersed systems (IUPAC recommendation. Pure Appl Chem 83:2229–2259
53. Larpent C et al (1997) Polymerization in microemulsions with polymerizable cosurfactants: a route to highly functionalized. Macromolecules 30:354–362
54. Mackay RA, Pileni MP, Moumen N (1999) Polymerization of methacrylate in WO microemulsion stabilized by a methacrylate surfactant. Coll Surf A 151:409–417
55. Capek I, Chern CS (2001) Mini-emulsions systems. Adv Polym Sci 155:101–165
56. Crespy D, Landfester K (2010) Miniemulsion polymerization as a versatile tool for the synthesis of functionalized polymers. Beilstein J Org Chem 6:1132–1148
57. Li TD et al (1996) Preparation of ultrafiltration membranes by direct miniemulsion polymerization using polymerizable surfactants. Langmuir 12:5863–5868
58. Wand HH (2010) Synthesis, morphology and rheology of core-shell silicone acrylic emulsion stabilized with polymerizable surfactant. eXPRESS Polym Lett 4:670–680
59. Zetterlund PB, Kagawa Y, Okubo M (2008) Controlled/living radical polymerization in dispersed systems. Chem Rev 108:3747–3794
60. Ringsdorf H, Thuning D (1977) On the kinetics of the polymerization of some ammonium methacrylates with different alkyl chain lengths in aqueous solution. Macromol Chem 178:2205–2210
61. Yegorov VV et al (1990) Study of structurization of in radical polymerization of cationic surface active monomers in toluene. Polym Sci USSR 32:2569–2575
62. Nagai K, Satoh H, Kuramoto N (1993) Polymerization of surface active monomers: 7. Radical copolymerizations of anionic surface active monomer, sodium di(10-undecenyl)sulfosuccinate, with electron-accepting monomers and vinyl monomers in micellar and isotropic solutions. Polymer 34:4969–4973
63. Pich A et al (2005) Polymeric particles prepared with fluorinated surfmer. Polymer 46:1323–1330
64. Cho HG et al (2010) Preparation and characterization of novel acrylic monomers. J Appl Polym Sci 116:736–742

65. Wang JS, Matyjascewski K (1995) Controlled/living radical polymerization. Halogen atom transfer radical polymerization promoted by Cu(I)/Cu(II) redox process. Macromolecules 28:7901–7910
66. Wang JS, Matyjascewski K (1995) Controlled/living radical polymerization. Atom transfer radical polymerization in the presence of transition-metal complexes. J Am Chem Soc 117:5614–5615
67. Kato M et al (1995) Polymerization of methyl methacrylate with the carbon tetrachloride/ dichlorotris-(triphenylphosphine)ruthenium(II)/ methylaluminum bis(2,6-di- tertbutylphenoxide) initiating system: possibility of living radical polymerization. Macromolecules 28:1721–1722
68. Braunecker WA, Matyjascewski K (2007) Controlled/living radical polymerization: features, developments, and perspectives. Prog Polym Sci 32:93–146
69. Min K et al (2009) One-pot synthesis of hairy nanoparticles by emulsion ATRP. Macromolecules 42:1597–1603
70. Dubois P et al (2006) Preparation of well defined poly[(ethylene oxide)- block—(sodium 2-acrylamido-2-methyl—1-propane—sulfonate)] diblock copolymers by water based atom transfer radical polymerization. Macromol Rapid Commun 27:1489–1494
71. Armes SP et al (2003) Direct synthesis of well defined quaternized homopolymers and diblock copolymers via ATRP in protic media. Macromolecules 36:8268–8275
72. Bortolamei N et al (2011) Controlled aqueous atom transfer radical polymerization with electrochemical generation of the active catalyst. Angew Chem Int Ed 50:11391–11394
73. Simakova A et al (2012) Aqueous AGET ATRP. Macromolecules 45:6371–6379
74. Li W, Matjaszewski K (2011) Cationic surface-active monomers as reactive surfactants for AGET Emulsion ATRP n–butyl methacrylate. Macromolecules 44:5578–5585
75. Yuan J, Antonietti M (2011) Poly(ionic liquid)s: polymers expanding classical property profiles. Polymers 52:1469–1482
76. Shen Y et al (2005) Atom transfer radical polymerization of styrenic ionic liquid monomers and carbon dioxide absorption of the polymerized ionic liquids. J Polym Sci, Part A: Polym Chem 43:1432–1443
77. Moad G, Rizzardo E, Thang SH (2010) Reversible addition fragmentation chain transfer (RAFT) polymerization. Mat Matters 5(1):2
78. Semsarilar M, Perrier S (2010) Green reversible addition fragmentation chain transfer (RAFT) polymerization. Nat Chem 2:811–820
79. Chefari J et al (1998) Living free radical polymerization by reversible addition chain transfer: the RAFT process. Macromolecules 31:5559–5562
80. Matahwa H, McLeary JB, Sanderson RD (2006) Comparative study of classical surfactants and polymerizable surfactants (surfmers) in the reversible addition fragmentation chain transfer mediated miniemulsion polymerization of styrene and methyl methacrylate. J Polym Sci, Part A: Polym Chem 44:427–442
81. McLeary JB, Klumperman B (2006) RAFT mediated polymerization in heterogeneous media. Soft Matter 2:45–53
82. FitzGerald PA et al (2013) The effect of degree of polymerization of intra- and interchain micellization of a tail type cationic polysoap. Soft Matter 9:2711–2716
83. Kotzev A, Laschewsky A, Rakotoaly RH (2001) Polymerizable surfactants and micellar polymers bearing fluorocarbon hydrophobic chains based on styrene. Macromol Chem Phys 202:2257–2267
84. Topp KA (2006) Cationic oligomeric surfactants: novel synthesis and characterization. Dissertation, The University of Sydney
85. Gnanou Y et al (2008) Synthesis by RAFT and ionic responsiveness copolymers based on ionic liquid monomer units. Macromolecules 41:6299–6308
86. Shen et al (2008) Synthesis and magnetic properties of comb-like polymeric complexes based on thiazol ring and ionic liquid. J Polym Sci, Part A: Polym Chem 46:5123–5132
87. Yuan J et al (2011) Euro Polym J. doi:10.1016/j.eurpolymj.2010.09.030
88. Yeole N, Hundiwale D, Jana T (2011) Synthesis of core-shell polystyrene nanoparticles by surfactant free emulsion polymerization using macro-RAFT agent. J Coll Inter Sci 354:506–510

89. Raj V, Kunnetheri S (2014) Nonconjugated polyelectrolyte as efficient fluorescence quencher and their applications as biosensors: polymer-polymer interaction. Analitical Chem. doi:10.1155/2014/841857
90. Petrak K (1986) Review: polyelectrolyte complexes in biomedical applications. J Bioact Compat Polym 1:202–219
91. Adamczak M et al (2012) Polyelectrolyte multilayer capsules with quantum dots for biomedical applications. Colloids Surf B Biointerfaces 90:211–216
92. Rosso F et al (2003) New polyelectrolyte hydrogels for biomedical application. Mater Sci Eng. doi:10.1016/S0928-4931(02)00290-4
93. Wu H, Kawaguchi S, Ito K (2004) Synthesis and polymerization of tale-type polymerizable surfactants and hydrophobic counter-anion induced association of polyelectrolytes. Coll Polym Sci 282:1365–1373
94. Paul GK, Indi SS, Ramakrishnan S (2004) Synthesis and vesicular polymerization of novel counter-ion polymerizable/crosslinkable surfactants. J Polym Sci: Part A: Polym Chem 42:5271–5283
95. Vincent B (2003) Flocculation in the mixtures of cationic polyelectrolytes and anionic surfactants. Adv Colloid Interface Sci 106:1–22

Chapter 4
Application of Surface Active Monomers and Polymers Containing Links of Surface Active Monomers

4.1 The Importance of Polymers of Biomedical Application

The main aim of application of surfmers was aimed on obtaining the various polymeric materials with improved properties. Nowadays, surface-active monomers are widely applied for the creation of non-toxic and biocompatible materials capable for specific interaction with cells. Nowadays, the research into polymers of biomedical application is one of the most actual topics in chemistry, physics, and polymer chemistry. Utilization of novel polymers as biomaterials has greatly impacted the advancement of modern medicine. With success in understanding of origins of many diseases including genetic understanding of diseases, polymers of biomedical application (or biopolymers) became essential part of modern researches in biology and medicine.

The saccharide and peptide fragments in copolymer structure could act as specific vectors defining therefore the possibility of interaction of these macromolecules with cell membranes [1]. Therefore, the polymeric carrier bearing conjugated drug substance after sorption on targeted biological object can penetrate through cell membrane due to endocytosis [2]. The biological tolerance of polymeric particles with functionalized surface makes them attractive prospects for application as markers of pathogenic cells and polymeric carriers for drugs and genes delivery. It is known that the progress of gene therapy depends also from development of required vectors (delivery systems) for transvection of DNA [3]. The corresponding systems have to possess low toxicity and efficiently overpass cell barriers providing the delivery of nucleic acid [4]. Moreover, the carriers must be non-mutagenic and non-immunogenic [5]. Non-viral carriers, which could easily prepared in satisfied amounts, seem to be more safe than viral carriers in the sense of immunogenicity [6]. The component part of non-viral carriers for delivery of nucleic acid consists of polymers bearing cationic fragments, namely synthetic polypetides, chitozane, and polyethylene amines. These compounds are capable for effective binding of DNA [7]. The characteristics of

M. Borzenkov and O. Hevus, *Surface Active Monomers*,
SpringerBriefs in Materials, DOI: 10.1007/978-3-319-08446-6_4

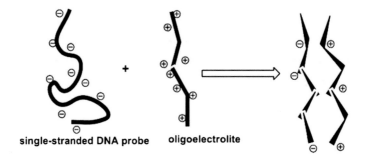

single-stranded DNA probe   oligoelectrolite

Scheme 4.1 The formation of oligoelectrolite–DNA complex

these polymers such as particle size, molecular weight, surface charge, and stability of polymer–DNA complex differently impact on transvection efficiency [8, 9]. The pH and ionic strength of medium essentially influence on structure and charge distribution in oligoelectrolite–DNA complexes [9]. For this purpose, the synthesis of new cationic surfmers with quaternary ammonium fragment seems to be the prospective way for creation of polymers for efficient binding of negatively charged biomolecules. Surface-active monomers with carboxylic groups are known to be prospective compounds for creation of anionic surface-active copolymers applied for drug delivery as well as for binding of peptides and amino acids [10]. Incorporation into the surfmer structure of more hydrophilic anionic fragment like a sulfonate group should improve the stability of complexes of copolymers containing links of surfmer with positively charged centers of biomolecules. The formation of oligoelectrolite–DNA complexes is schematically shown on Scheme 4.1.

From the other hand, non-ionic surfactant vesicles (niosomes) formed from self-assembly of hydrated synthetic non-ionic surface-active monomers and polymers with links of non-ionic surfmers are capable of entrapping a wide range of drugs and were evaluated as an alternative to liposomes [11]. In niosomes, soluble drug molecules are present in the aqueous compartments between the bilayer, whereas insoluble ones are entrapped within the bilayer matrix. The application of niosomes for drug delivery provides a greater degree of targeting of the drug to selected tissues, sustained release, and altered pharmacokinetics [12–14]. The simple structure of micelle of surface-active polymer with conjugated drug is shown on Scheme 4.2.

Also, the attention is focused on developing of new materials for manufacturing medical devices, dental composites, and scaffolds for tissue engineering [15–17].

Summarizing this, it should be concluded that in recent years, polymers have been tailored for specific biomedical and pharmaceutical applications starting with new and designed monomers expanding to specific and controlled polymerizations that allow for tightly controlling molar masses and molar mass distributions [18]. A short overview about biomedical application of surface-active monomers and polymers containing units of surfmers is done.

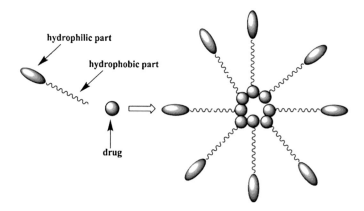

Scheme 4.2 Simple scheme of micelle with conjugated drug

4.2 The Application of Surfmers for Creating Materials of Biomedical Application. A Brief Review of Publications

The application of surface-active monomer, polyisobutylene-succinimide pentamine (Lubrizol U) as a stabilizer for synthesizing polyurea nanocapsules with aqueous core via polyaddition at inverse miniemulsion droplet interface was reported in the paper published in Langmuir in 2009 [19]. Due to the presence of amine groups in the Lubrizol molecule, it is covalently incorporated into the polymeric interfacial layer after reaction, resulting in more compact capsule shell. As an example for biomedical application, the fluorescein-containing capsules were utilized in cell uptake experiments and visualized using fluorescence microscopy. The utilization of fumaric-, maleic-, and itaconic reactive surface-active monomer with fluorine containing groups for manufacturing of materials which can be usefully employed for the fabrication of prostheses such as heart valves and intraocular lenses, as optical contact lenses or as films, was claimed in US patent published in 2009 [15]. The incorporation of nitrogen-containing monomers, especially surface active, to the main chain or side chain of polymers opens wide opportunities of obtaining materials with a range of improved properties [20]. Therefore, the utilization of such monomers for obtaining the latexes of biomedical application became an attractive and prospective issue. Such latexes could be applied for immunodiagnostic systems, manufacturing of contact lenses, treatment of some diseases, for example silicosis, binding of enzymes and microorganisms, and coating of drugs [20]. For this purpose, the grafting of 4-(diethylamino) butylacrylate to the surface of polystyrene latex particles aimed on obtaining of creation of polymeric base for antibody carrier for novel immunodiagnostic systems was carried out [21]. It was found that resulted carrier was capable for chemisorption of α-chemotripsine proteins, IgG antibodies of human immunoglobuline in amount 0.3 mg per 1 mg of dry polymer that was corresponded to a protein monolayer [21].

In the introduction, it was stated that surface-active monomers containing the fragment of compounds of nature origin or with biosurfactant moieties nowadays are essential of creation of novel classes of materials of biomedical application. In addition, biosurfactants present several advantages over synthetic surfactants connected with their biodegradability, low toxicity, and high selectivity and specific activity at extreme temperatures, pH, and salinity [22, 23]. The recently published review focuses on the most recent biomedical and therapeutic applications of biosurfactants with emphasis on the most recent results in the fields of biotechnology, nanotechnology, and bioengineering [24]. Latex particles bearing carbohydrate species were prepared by emulsion copolymerization of styrene or methyl methacrylate with polymerizable liposaccharide surfactants [25]. The potential application of these functionalized latexes in the biomedical diagnostic field was evaluated by studying the adsorption of bovine serum albumin, and by performing covalent binding of antibodies and single-stranded DNA fragments on their surface.

The surface-active monomers synthesized from pyromellitic dianhydride and glycerol dimethacrylate were applied for adhesive bonding of dentin [26]. The application of polymers based on bis(vinylcyclopropane) and bis(methacrylate) monomers with cholesteryl group for dental composites was reported in paper published in 2013 [16]. The synthesis of the cyclodextrin derivatives and derived polymers capable for bonding of hydrolytically stable polymers to dental and perhaps other biological tissues was reported [27].

Graft polymerization of N,N'-dimethyl-N-methacryloyloxyethyl-N-(3-sulfopropyl) ammonium, a zwitterionic sulfobetaine structure monomer, onto the ozone-activated silicone surface was performed [28]. The blood compatibility of the grafted films was evaluated by platelet adhesion in platelet-rich plasma and protein adsorption in bovine fibrinogen using silicone film as the reference. The protein adsorption was reduced on the grafted films after incubated in bovine fibrinogen for 120 min. These results confirmed that the improved blood compatibility was obtained by grafting this new zwitterronic sulfobetaine structure onto silicone film.

It is known that compounds containing quaternary ammonium fragment possess bactericidal properties [29]. Antibacterial and antifungal polymer brushes of alkylated 2-(dimethylamino)ethylmethacrylate were synthesized via controlled polymerization methods by Russel and coworkers [30, 31]. Palermo et al. [32] reported interesting results regarding the interaction of copolymer containing primary, secondary, and quaternary amine fragments with model membrane systems. They found that careful fine-tuning of the hydrophobic and hydrophilic groups increased the pronounced interactions of the polymers with biomembranes, including possible amine-phosphate complexation after initial binding of the polymer to the membrane [33]. The antimicrobial properties of (dimethylamino)ethylmethacrylate derivatives with varying spacer and alkyl chain lengths were investigated [34]. Novel, non-leaching bioactive nanoparticles polystyrene nanoparticles were synthesized by introducing quaternized (dimethylamino) ethylmethacrylate surface-active comonomers capable for stabilizing colloidal system as well as providing biological quaternary ammonium moieties to the resulting nanoparticles surface [33]. The biological studies indicated the potential of resulted nanoparticles as promising bactericidal contact-active agents.

A tutorial review of Park et al. [35] provides an overview of polymeric self-assembled monolayers of various types of surface-active copolymers. It also discusses design principles for polymeric self-assembled monolayers to tune interfacial and surface interactions of materials for potential biomedical applications. The application of various self-assembled monomers and oligomers with at least one reactive chemical group capable of binding them to the terminus of a polymer, modifying end group of that polymer, was described in US patent published in 2012 [36]. These polymers could be successfully applied for construction of medical and drug delivery devices.

Nelson [37] and coworkers studied the addition of thiol-containing amino acids to surface-active monoalkkyl maleic salts. However, maleimide containing monomers as Michael acceptors are considered to be more favorable compounds for binding of thiol groups forming stable thioether bonds [38]. The technique of binding the peptides of gonadortropins (or glycoproteine hormones) by macromolecular carriers synthesized on the basis of maleimide containing compounds was developed [39]. A new strategy for functionalizing the ω-terminal end of polymers synthesized by reversible addition–fragmentation chain transfer polymerization that provides spatially controlled bioconjugation sites was described [40]. This technique was demonstrated the utilization of N-(2-aminoethyl)maleimide trifluoroacetate to introduce a single primary amine to the ω-terminus of poly(dimethy-laminoethyl methacrylate) and poly(N-isopropyl acrylamide) and to a specialized block copolymer for siRNA delivery. The versatile chain-extension technique described in this paper offers opportunities for the synthesis of well-defined polymeric conjugates to molecules of biological and targeting interest. Modified supramolecular aggregates for selective delivery of contrast agents and/or drugs were examined with a focus on a new class of peptide-derivatized nanoparticles: naposomes. These nanoparticles are based on the co-aggregation of two different amphiphilic monomers that give aggregates of different shapes and sizes (micelles, vesicles, and liposomes) with diameters ranging between 10 and 300 nm [41]. The reported in the first chapter surface-active monomer, distearyl-phosphatidyl-ethalilamino-PEG$_{5000}$-maleimide was successfully applied for creation of novel and efficient drug carriers. The efficiency of surface-exposed peptides in homing these nanovectors to a specific target introduces promising new opportunities for the development of diagnostic and therapeutic agents with high specificity toward the biological target and reduced toxic side effects on non-target organs [41].

Phospholipid polymers are used for binding of various biomolecules such as proteins, peptides, and DNA [42, 43]. Therefore, Ishihara et al. [44] synthesized the monomer with phospholipid polar group, 2-methacryloyloxy phosphorylcholine, for obtaining polymeric structures of cell membranes. Another phospholipid polymer for bioconjugating was synthesized by copolymerization of 2-methacryloyloxy phosphorylcholine with n-nitrophenyloxycarbonyl(oxyethylene) methacrylate and n-butylmetacrylate [45].

A number of colloidal structures used in drug delivery formulations are described in detail in the review of Santos [46]. The properties and application of environment-sensitive hydrogels with cationic or anionic moieties as drugs carriers were described in review published in 2001 [47]. The application of polymers including polymers synthesized from surface-active monomers for mucoadhesive drug delivery system is described in a brief note published in 2009 [48]. Anionic polymeric network containing carboxylic or sulphonic acid groups could be used in the design of intelligent-controlled release devices for site-specific drug delivery of therapeutic proteins to large intestine, where the biological activity of the proteins is prolonged [49]. Hydrogels of poly(methyl methacrylate-co-dimethylaminoethyl methacrylate) were studied for diffusion coefficients of different water-soluble drugs [50]. Cationic hydrogels are used in the preparation of self-regulated insulin delivery systems [51]. The use of cationic hydrogels in the preparation of self-regulated insulin delivery systems was reviewed in the publication of Shivakumar and Satish [52]. Commercially available, reactive hydrophilic, sulfonic acid acrylic monomer, 2-acrylamido-2-methylpropane sulfonic acid (AMPS), due to the range of important properties, is widely used for the preparation of anionic polymers of biomedical application [53, 54]. As a good hydrophilic monomer, AMPS is used for the preparation of superabsorbent hydrogels which is known to be useful in various fields including pharmaceuticals [55, 56].

A small library of novel multifunctional small interfering RNA carriers, polymerizable surfactants with pH-sensitive amphiphilicity based on the hypothesis that pH-sensitive amphiphilicity and environmentally sensitive small interfering RNA release can result in efficient small interfering RNA delivery was reported [57]. The polymerizable surfactants comprise a protonatable amino head group, two cysteine residues, and two lipophilic tails. The corresponding surfactants demonstrated pH-sensitive amphiphilic hemolytic activity or cell membrane disruption with rat red blood cells. The utilization of novel lipids comprise polymerizable linkers and surfactants that can link "targeting" molecules to the surface of drug delivery systems and facilitate drug uptake across mucosal surfaces was described in US patent published in 1999 [58].

A variety of non-viral delivery vectors were developed such as polymers and surfactants [59]. As a result, polymerizable surfactants with tunable pH-sensitive amphiphilicity have been developed recently. These properties allow carriers to change their amphiphilic structure at endosomal-lyposomal pH resulted in distribution endosomal-lyposomal membranes [58–60]. A tellurium-based polymeric surfactant as a seleno-enzyme model has been constructed by employing 11-acryloyloxyundecyltriethylammonium bromide and a tellurium-containing compound [61]. It demonstrates strong substrate-binding ability for thiols and high glutathione peroxidase (GPx) activity. A series of tellurium-based polymeric micelle catalysts with the catalytic tellurium center located at various positions in the micelle were designed. The publication of Garay-Jimenez [62] and coworkers summarizes their investigations of poly(butyl acrylate-styrene) emulsions made using anionic, cationic, zwitterionic, and non-charged (amphiphilic) surfactants, as well as attachable surfactant monomers comparing the cytotoxicity and microbiological activity levels of the emulsions. Incorporation of an N-thiolated β-lactam antibacterial agent onto the nanoparticle matrix via covalent attachment endows the emulsion with antibiotic properties against pathogenic bacteria such as methicillin-resistant Staphylococcus aureus, without changing the physical properties of the nanoparticles or their emulsions.

In the Chap. 1, it was told about the significant biomedical importance of surfmers bearing maleimide group as maleimide group can facilitate covalent attachment of proteins and other molecules to polymers. Moreover, compounds containing maleimide and PEG fragments are successfully applied for monitoring of release, biodistribution, toxicology of drugs, and proteins. Novel surface-active monomer distearyl-phosphatidyl–ethanilamino-PEG$_{5000}$-maleimide was synthesized and successfully applied for design of efficient carriers of the drugs [63]. In vitro and in vivo behaviors of these carriers were discussed. The new carriers could promote promising opportunities for the development of diagnostic and therapeutic agents with high specificity toward the biological target and reduced toxic side effects on nontarget organs. Photon-upconverting nanoparticles have become an important new class of optical labels. Their unique property of emitting visible light after photo-excitation with near-infrared radiation enables biological imaging without background interference or cell damage. In the paper published in 2012, three different types of maleimide-functionalized photon-upconverting nanoparticles were prepared and characterized by transmission electron microscopy, dynamic light scattering and Raman spectroscopy [64]. Ligand exchange of oleic acid by maleimide–PEG–COOH yielded to nanoparticles that did not aggregate, were colloidally stable and reacted readily with proteins. Such luminescent labels are required for background-free imaging and many other bioanalytical applications.

Another way of application of surface-active polymers derived of surface-active monomers is a coating of metal and metal oxide nanoparticles for biomedical purposes. These systems could be considered as promising nanovectors for targeted curing of cancer without the use of drugs. For this matter, two therapies are studied: hyperthermia and photothermal therapy. In the first one, superparamagnetic material is accumulated on the tumor site; then, the application of an alternated magnetic field causes heating in the range of 41–47 °C, provoking preferential death of cancerous cells while sparing healthy cells, while in the second one, precious metal is accumulated on the tumor site; then, the application of a near-infrared irradiation causes heating in the range of 41–47 °C, provoking preferential death of cancerous cells while sparing healthy cells [65–67]. Moreover, in order to be suitable for intravenous administration, these nanovectors need to be biocompatible and further functionalized for active targeting.

At the end of this chapter, it should be said that the biomedical application of surface-active monomers was briefly described. However, nowadays, there is huge amount of publications focused on current topic. This could serve as evidence of significant importance of utilizing a variety of special surface-active monomers and polymers for solving actual problems in the field of medicine and biology.

References

1. Nickels JD, Schmidt CE (2013) Surface modification of the conductive polymer, polypyrroole, via affinity peptide. J Biomed Mater Res A 101:1464–1471
2. Lee J et al (2013) Caveolae-mediated endocytosis of conjugated polymer nanoparticles. Macromol Biosci 13:913–920

3. Patil SD, Rhodes DG, Burgess DJ (2004) Anionic liposomal delivery system for DNA transfection. AAPS J 6:13–22
4. Luo D, Salzman WM (2003) Synthetic dna delivery systems. Kluwer Academic, New York
5. Liu D, Chia EF, Tian H (2003) Chemical methods of DNA delivery: an overview. Methods Mol Biol 245:3–23
6. Brown MD, Schatzlein AG, Uchegbu IF (2001) Gene delivery with synthetic (non-viral) carriers. Int J Pharm 229:1–21
7. Mänisto M (2007) Polymeric carriers in non-viral gene delivery. Dissertation, University of Kuopio
8. Zhang X et al (2006) Physicochemical properties of low molecular weight alkylated chitosans: a new class of potential nonviral vectors for gene delivery. Colloids Surf B Biointerfaces 51:140–148
9. Zaichenko A et al (2008) Development of novel linear, block and branched oligoelectrolytes and functionally targeting nanoparticles. Pure Appl Chem 80:2309–2326
10. Tang MX, Szoka FC (1997) The influence of polymer structure on the interactions of cationic polymers with DNA and morphology of the resulting complexes. Gene Ther 8:823–832
11. Florence AT, Bailie AJ (1989) Non-ionic surfactant vesicles: alternatives to liposomes in drug delivery. In: Prescot LF, Nimmo WS (eds) Novel drug delivery and its therapeutic applications. Wiley, Chichester
12. Florence AT et al (1990) Non-ionic surfactant vesicles as carriers of doxorubicin. In: Gregoriadis G (ed) Targeting of drugs. Plenum, New York
13. Chandraprakash KS et al (1993) Effect of niosome encapsulation of methotrexate, macrophage activation, and tissue distribution of methotrexate and tumor size. Drug Deliv 1:333–337
14. Kandasamy R, Vientramuthu S (2010) Formulation and optimization of zidovudine niosomes. AAPS Pharm Sci Tech 11:1119–1127
15. Weihong L, Lai YC (2009) Novel polymerizable surface active monomers with both fluorine-containing groups and hydrophilic groups. US Patent 8071704 B2, 9 Apr 2009
16. Choi SW (2013) Bis(vinylcyclopropane) and bis(methacrylate) monomers with cholesteryl group for dental composites. e-Polymers 5:820–831
17. Wang S et al (2010) Surface modification of polymers via surface active and reactive end groups. US patent WO2010057080 A1, 10 March 2010
18. Scholz C, Kressler J (2013) In tailored polymer architectures for pharmaceutical and biomedical applications. ACS Symposium Series, Washington DC
19. Rosenbauer EM, Landfester K, Musyanovych A (2009) Surface active monomer as a stabilizer for polyurea nanocapsules synthesized via interfacial polyaddition in inverse miniemulsion. Langmuir 25:12084–12091
20. Kameya M, Yoshida T (1989) Water soluble monomers. Kobunshi Kako 38:398–409
21. Kohut AM (2006) Sintez i vlastuvosti poverhnevo-aktuvnuh monomeriv i peroxydiv (Synthesis and properties of surface active monomers and peroxides). Dissertation, Lviv Polytechnic National University
22. Banat IM (1995) Biosurfactants production and use in microbial enhanced oil recovery and pollution remediation: a review. Bioresour Technol 51:1–12
23. Banat IM et al (2010) Microbial biosurfactants production, applications and future potential. Appl Microbiol Biotechnol 87:427–444
24. Fracchia L et al (2012) Biosurfactants and bioemulsifiers biomedical and related applications—present status and future potential. In: Ghista DN (ed) Biomedical Science, Engineering and Technology, Chapter 14
25. Charreyere MT et al (1999) Surface functionalization of polystyrene nanoparticles with liposaccharide monomers: preparation, characterization and application. J Bioact Compatible Polym 14:64–90
26. Venz S, Dickens B (1993) Modified surface active polymers for adhesive bonding of dentin. J Dent Res 72:582
27. Bowen RL (2009) Synthesis of polymerizable cyclodextrin derivatives for use in adhesion-promoting monomer formulations. J Res Natl Ins Stand Technol 114:1–9

28. Youling Y et al (2003) Grafting sulfobetaine monomer onto silicone surface to improve haemocompatibility. Polym Int 53:121–126
29. Isquitz AJ, Walters PA (1972) Surface-bonded antimicrobial activity of an organosilicon quaternary ammonium chloride. Appl Microbiol 24:859–863
30. Ravikumar T et al (2006) Surface active antifungal polyquarternary amine. Biomacromolecules 7:2762–2769
31. Murata H et al (2007) Permanent, non-leaching, antibacterial surfaces – 2: How high density cationic surfaces kill bacterial cells. Biomaterials 28:4870–4879
32. Palermo EF et al (2011) Role of cationic group structure in membrane binding and disruption by amphiphilic copolymers. J Phys Chem B 115:366–375
33. Schwartz VB (2011) Design of nanoparticles systems with antimicrobial properties. Dissertation, Johannes Gutenberg-Universität Mainz
34. Caillier at al (2009) Synthesis and antimicrobial properties of polymerizable quaternary ammoniums. Eur j Med Chem 44:3201–3208
35. Park JW, Kim H, Han M (2010) Polymeric self-assembled monolayers derived from surface-active copolymers: a modular approach to functionalized surfaces. Chem Soc Rev 39:2935–2947
36. Ward SR et al (2012) Self-assembling monomers and oligomers as surface-modifying endgroups of polymers. US patent 20120095166, 19 Apr 2012
37. Nilson K et al (2007) Addition of thiol containing ligands to surface active Michael acceptor. Macromolecules 40:901–908
38. Trivedi B (1982) Maleic anhydride. Culberston, New York
39. Lee CJ et al (1980) A method for preparing β-hCG COOH peptide-carrier conjugates of predictable composition. Mol Immunol 17:749–756
40. Scott MH, Convertine AJ, Danielle S (2009) End-functionalized polymers and junction-functionalized diblock copolymers VIA RAFT chain extension with maleimdo monomers. Bioconjugate Chem 20:1122–1128
41. Accardo A et al (2011) Naposomes: a new class of peptide-derivatized, target-selective multimodal nanoparticles
42. Ishihara K et al (2004) A water soluble phospholipid polymer as a new biocompatible synthetic DNA carrier. Bull Chem Soc Jpn 77:2283–2288
43. Palmer RR et al (2004) Biologica evaluation and drug delivery application of cationically modified phospholipid polymers. Biomaterials 19:4785–4796
44. Ishihara K et al (2006) Water structure and improved mechanical properties of phospholipid polymer hydrogel with phosphorylcholine centered intermolecular cross-linker. Polymer 47:1390
45. Ishihara K et al (2006) UCST-type cononosolvency behavior of poly (2-methacryloxyethyl phosphorylcholine) in the mixture of water and ethanol. Polym J 40:479–483
46. Santos S et al (2013) Amphiphilic molecules in drug delivery systems. In: Coelho J (ed) Drug delivery systems: advanced technologies potentially applicable in personalised treatment
47. Qui Y, Park K (2001) Environment-sensitive hydrogels for drug delivery. Adv Drug Deliv Rev 53:321–339
48. Roy S et al (2009) Polymers in mucoadhesive drug delivery systems: A brief note. Des Monomers Polym 12:483–495
49. Lugo MT, Peppas NA (1999) Molecular design and in vitro studies of novel pH-sensitive hydrogels for the oral delivery of calcitonin. Macromolecules 32:6646–6651
50. Varshosaz J, Falamarzian M (2001) Drug diffusion mechanism through pH-sensitive hydrophobic/polyelectrolyte hydrogel membranes. Eur J Pharm Biopharm 51:235–240
51. Satish CS, Satish KP, Shivakumar HG (2006) Hydrogels as controlled drug delivery systems: synthesis, crosslinking, water and drug transport mechanism. Indian J Pharm Sci 68:133–140
52. Shivakumar HG, Satish CS (2004) Recent developments in self-regulated insulin delivery. Indian J Pharm Sci 66:137–141
53. Ogawa M et al (2012) Poly(2-acrylamido-2-methylpropanesulfonic acid) gel induces articular cartilage regeneration in vivo: Comparison of the induction ability between single- and double-network gels. J Biomed Mat Res Part A 100A:2244–2251

54. Ottenbrite RM (2010) Biomedical applications of hydrogels handbook. Springer, New York
55. Wang Y et al (2013) Synthesis, characterization, and swelling behaviors of a pH-responsive CMC-g-poly(AA-co-AMPS) superabsorbent hydrogel. Turk J Chem 37:149–159
56. Bao Y, Ma JZ, Li N (2011) Synthesis and swelling behaviors of sodium carboxymethyl cellulose-g-poly(AA-co-AM-co-AMPS)/ montmorillonite superabsorbent hydrogel. Carbohydr Polym 84:76–82
57. Wang XL et al (2007) Novel polymerizable surfactants with pH-sensitive amphiphilicity and cell membrane disruption for efficient siRNA delivery. Bioconjug Chem 18:2169–2177
58. Brey NR, Liang L (1999) Novel polymerizable fatty acids, phospholipids and polymerized liposomes made therefrom. US patent WO 1999033940 A1, 8 July 1999
59. Nogueira DR et al (2011) The role of the concentrations in the membrane-disruptive properties of pH-sensitive lysine based surfactants. Acta Biomater 7:2846–2856
60. Wang XL et al (2008) A multifunctional and reversible polymerizable carrier for efficient siRNA delivery. Biomaterials 29:15–22
61. Huang X et al (2006) Tellurium-based polymeric surfactants as a novel seleno-enzyme model with high activity. Macromol Rapid Commun 27:2101–2106
62. Garay-Jimenez JC et al (2009) Physical properties and biological activity of poly(butyl acrylate-styrene) nanoparticles emulsions prepared with conventional and polymerizable surfactants. Nanomed: Nanotechnol, Biol Med 5:443–451
63. Accardo A et al (2011) Naposomes : a new class of peptide-derivatized, poly(butyl acrylate-styrene) nanoparticles target-selective multimodal nanoparticles for imaging therapeutic applications. Ther Delivery 2:235–257
64. Liebher RB et al (2012) Maleimide activation of photon upconverting nanoparticles for bioconjugation. Nanotechnology 23, doi: 10.1088/0957-4484/23/48/485103
65. Amici J et al (2011) Poly(ethylene glycol)-coated magnetite nanoparticles: preparation and characterization. Macromol Chem Phys 212:6. doi:10.1002/macp.201000707
66. Amici J et al (2012) Polymer grafting onto magnetite nanoparticles by "click" reaction. J Mater Sci, Springer 47:8. doi:10.1007/s10853-011-5814-z
67. Amici J et al (2011) Photochemical synthesis of gold- polyethylenglycol core-shell nanoparticles. Eur Polym J 47:6. doi:10.1016/j.europolymj.2011.03.007

Conclusions

Surface active monomers due to their amphiphilicity, presence of polymerizable fragments and (in many cases) various functional groups are considered to be essential for creation of polymeric colloidal systems with a range of valuable and important properties. This review briefly highlighted the main aspects connected with surface active monomers, namely their synthesis, colloidal and polymerization properties and application. The emphasis has been done on the application of the corresponding compounds for current and emerge needs of medicine, biology and pharmacy.

© The Author(s) 2014
M. Borzenkov and O. Hevus, *Surface Active Monomers*,
SpringerBriefs in Materials, DOI: 10.1007/978-3-319-08446-6